Current Topics on Military Medicine

Edited by Nikolai V. Gorbunov

Published in London, United Kingdom

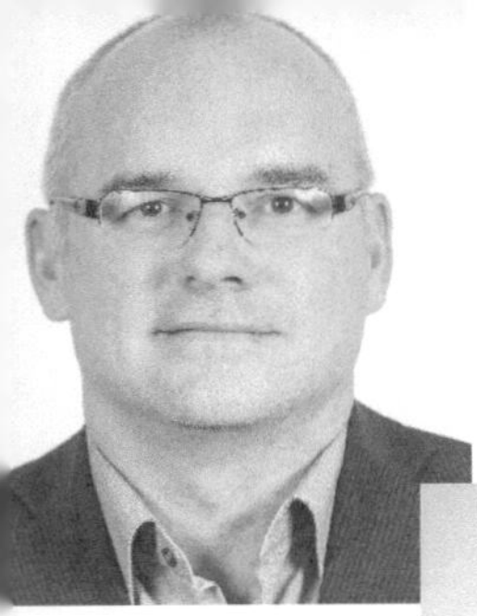
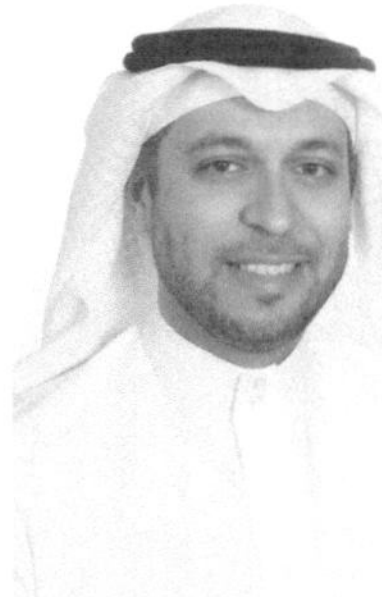
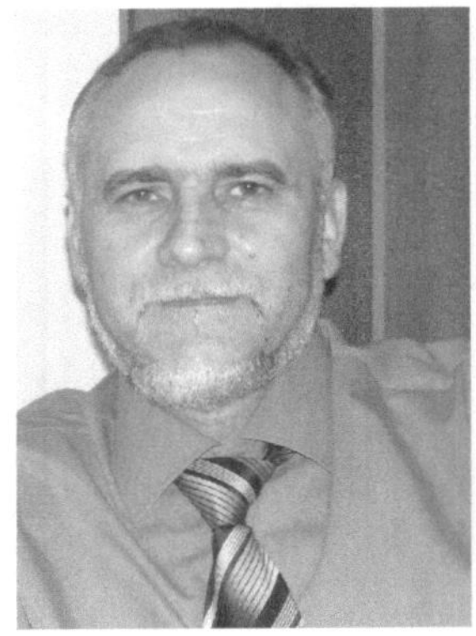
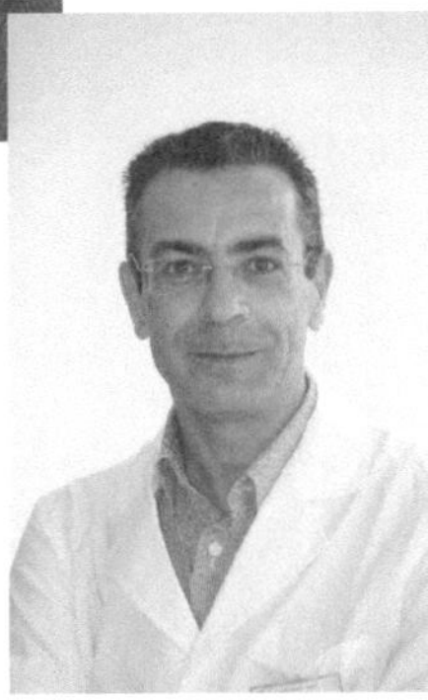
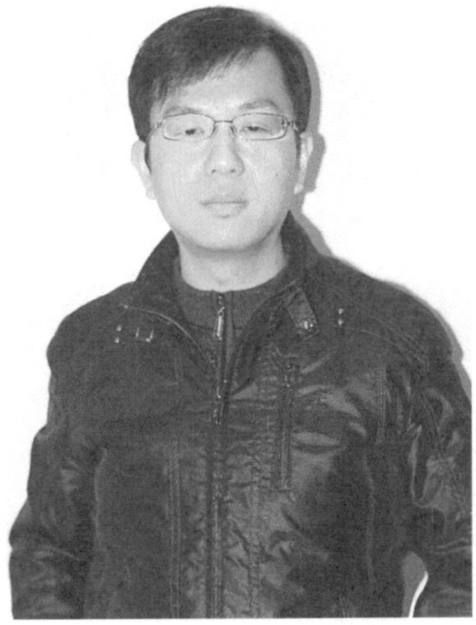
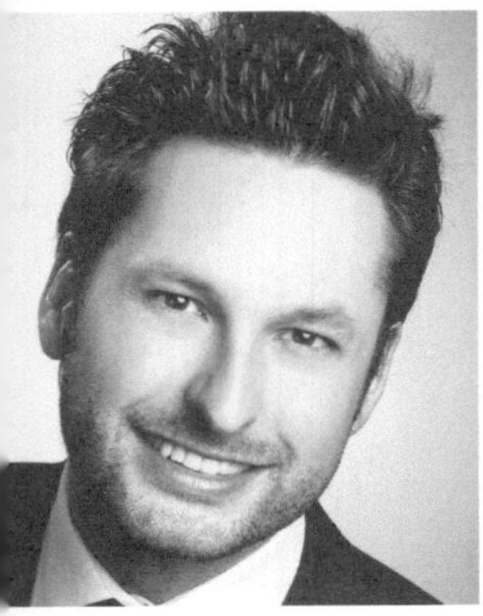
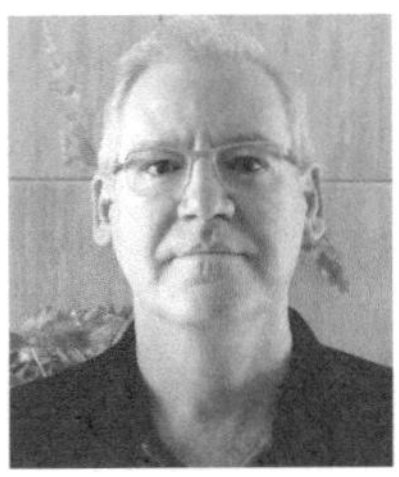

IntechOpen

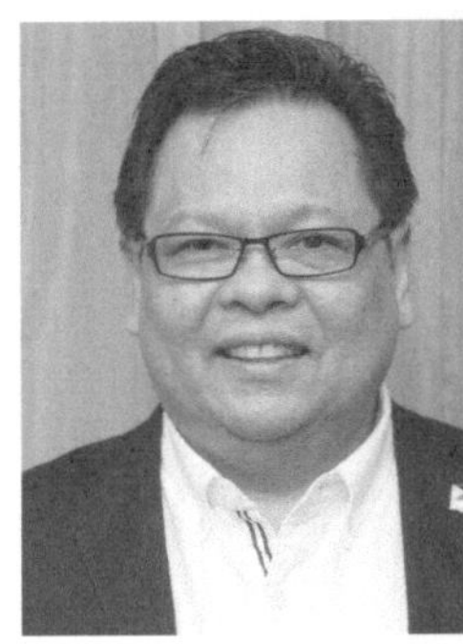
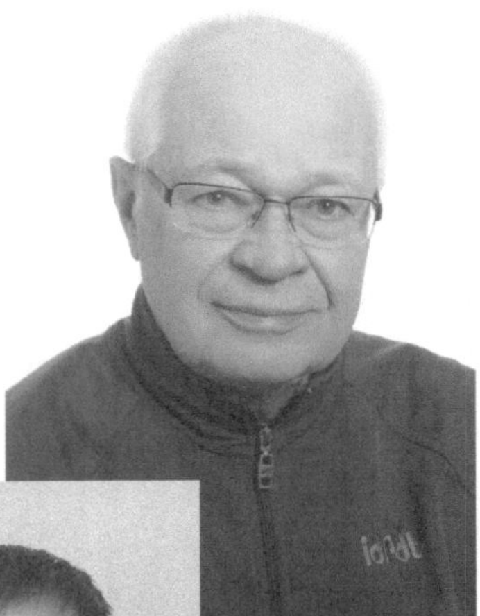
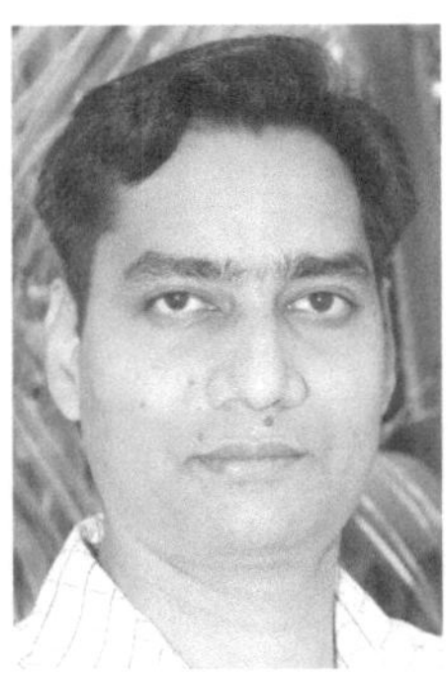
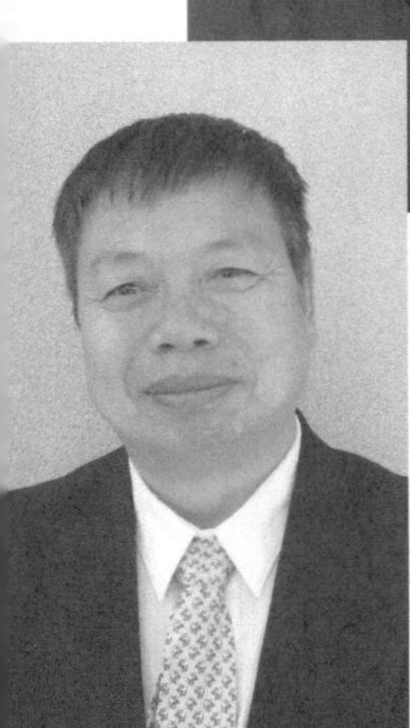
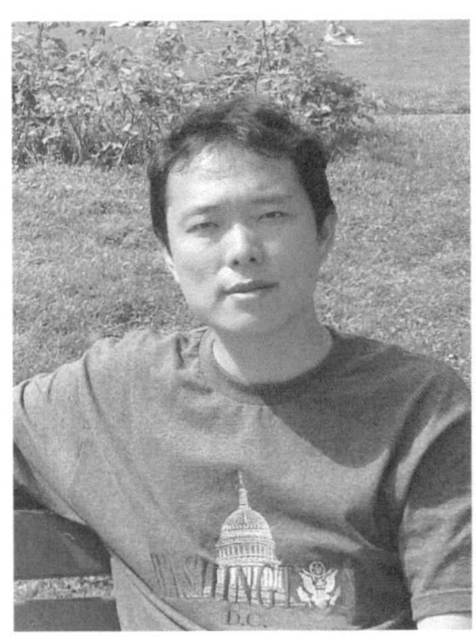
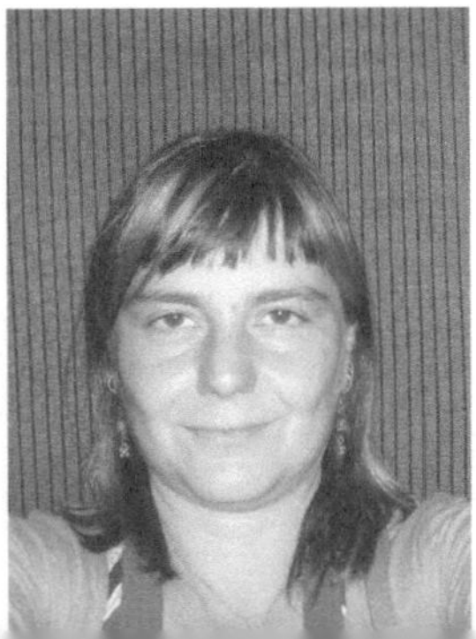

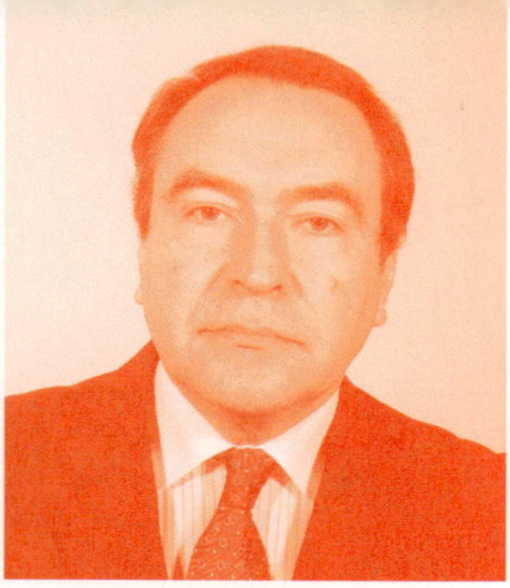
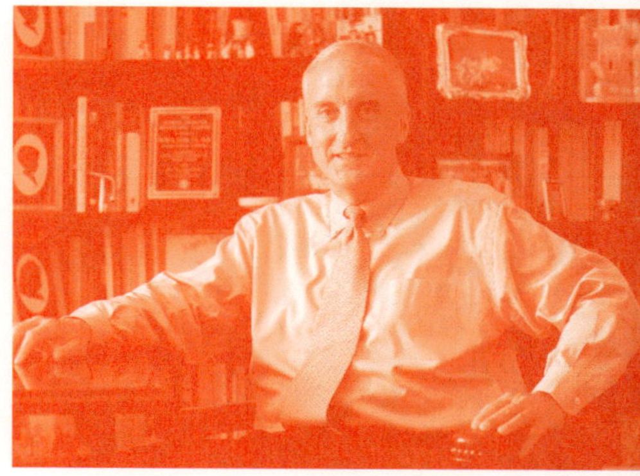
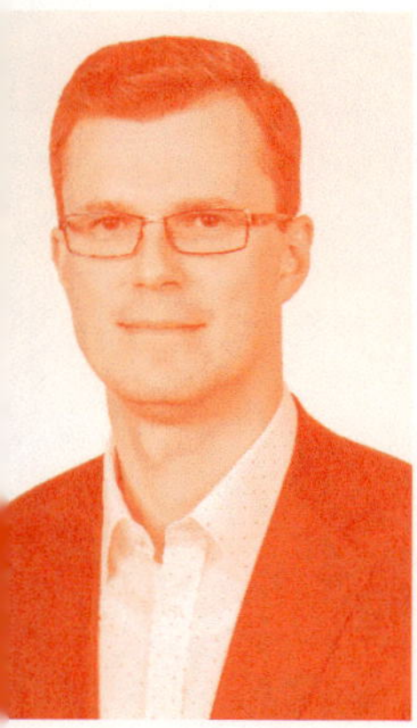
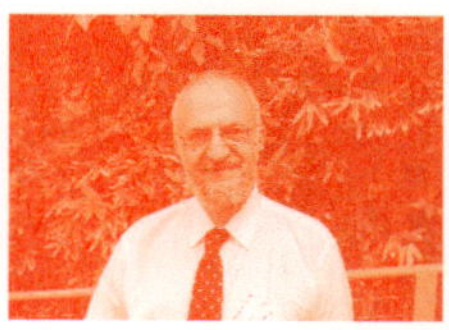
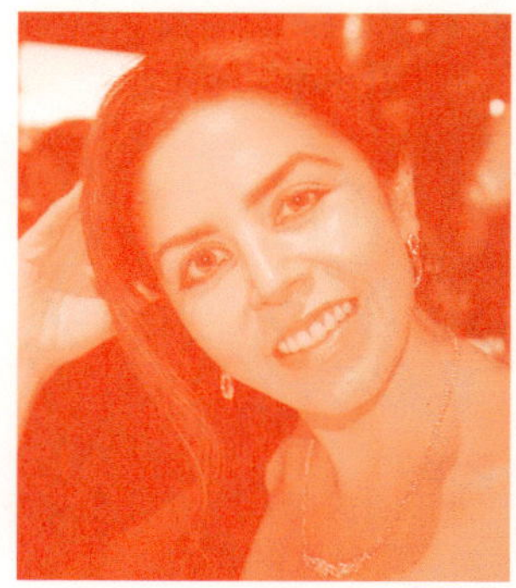

Supporting open minds since 2005

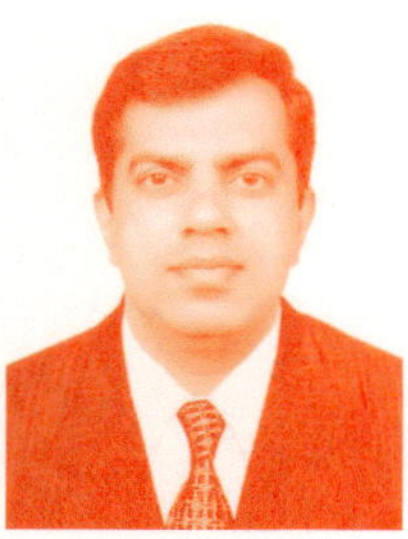
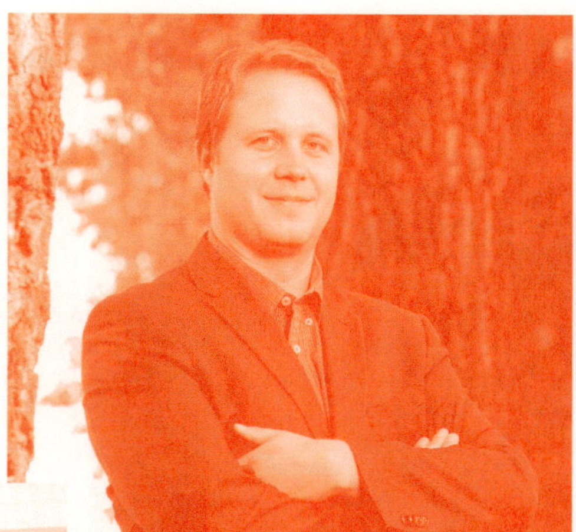
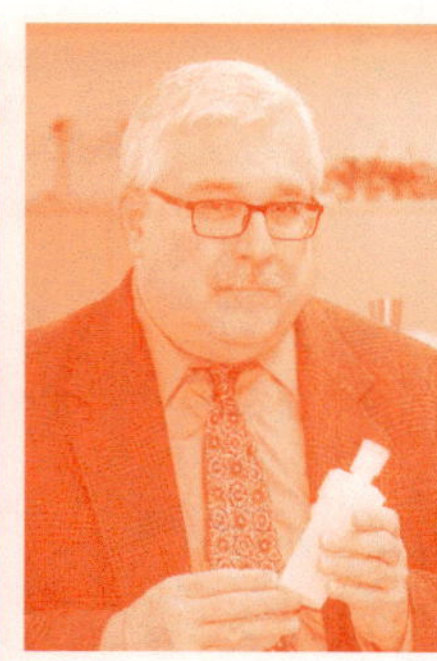
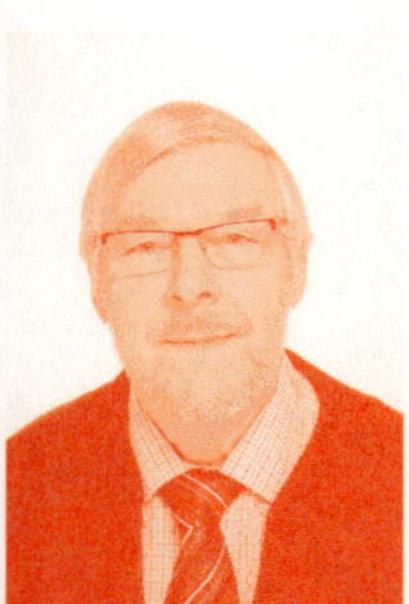
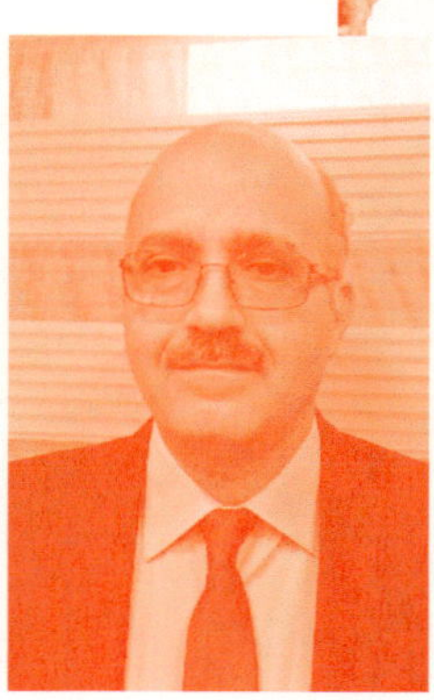
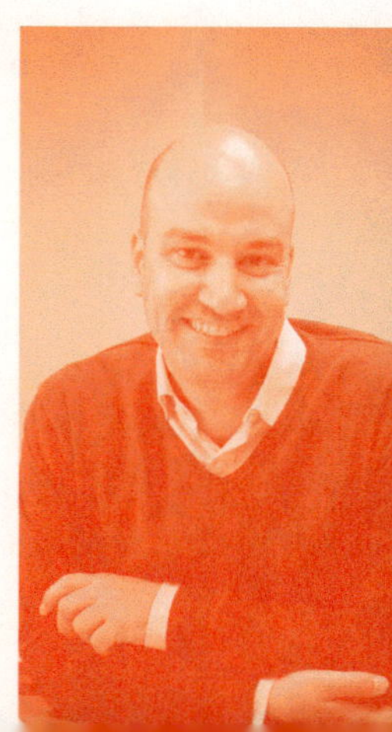
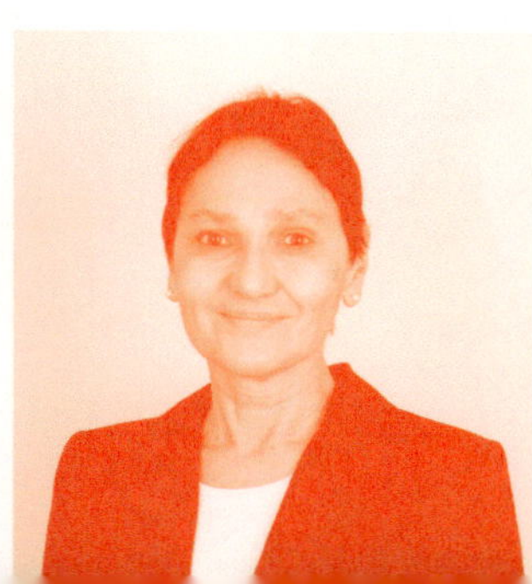

Current Topics on Military Medicine
http://dx.doi.org/10.5772/intechopen.87358
Edited by Nikolai V. Gorbunov

Contributors
Sunil Jain, Lei Zhang, Robert Ursano, Xianzhang Hu, Xiaoxia Li, Alan L. Peterson, Barbara L. Niles, Stacey Young-McCaughan, Terence M. Keane, Abhishek Kadian, Sachin Saini, Rajesh Khanna, Nikolai Gorbunov

First published in London, United Kingdom, 2021 by IntechOpen
IntechOpen is the global imprint of INTECHOPEN LIMITED, registered in England and Wales, registration number: 11086078, 5 Princes Gate Court, London, SW7 2QJ, United Kingdom
Printed in Croatia

British Library Cataloguing-in-Publication Data
A catalogue record for this book is available from the British Library

Additional hard and PDF copies can be obtained from orders@intechopen.com

Current Topics on Military Medicine
Edited by Nikolai V. Gorbunov
p. cm.
Print ISBN 978-1-83968-994-9
Online ISBN 978-1-83968-995-6
eBook (PDF) ISBN 978-1-83968-996-3

Meet the editor

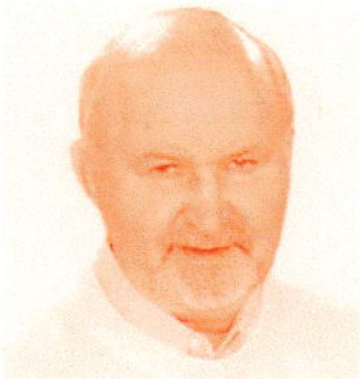

Dr. Nikolai V. Gorbunov received a Ph.D. in Biology from the Russian Academy of Sciences. He was granted a postdoctoral research award by the NRC Research Associateship Programs, after which he joined the Walter Reed Army Institute of Research (WRAIR), Maryland, USA, to pursue postdoctoral training and research on biophysics and molecular and cellular pathology of blast-related polytrauma. Dr. Gorbunov completed a DoE-sponsored training in radiation sciences and radiation health at the University of Pittsburgh and the Pacific Northwest National Laboratory, Washington, USA (www.emsl.pnl.gov/emslweb). His translational research areas include redox homeostasis, cellular mechanisms of barrier functions in conjunction with the biology of blast polytrauma, and acute radiation illness. In this framework, he investigated molecular and cellular mechanisms leading to vascular dysfunction and impairment of tissue barriers in the pathogenesis of radiation-combined injury with a focus on the development of new remedies for the management of the diseases. He conducted this research at WRAIR and the Uniformed Services University of the Health Sciences, Maryland, USA (https://www.usuhs.edu).

Contents

Preface

The tremendous social, economic and technological development of modern societies has created a global civilization, yet the threat of military force with conventional weapon systems, weapons of mass destruction, and weaponized machinery remains an indispensable tactical approach in pursuing the "doctrine of national interests" on land and sea and, recently, in air and space.

However, therein lies the fundamental problems in the recent era of combat operations: despite advanced training, personal protection, and even human enhancements, human frailty is unavoidable, as is the risk of complex adverse health outcomes in warfighters. Along with this, there is a devastating toll of the direct and ancillary effects of traumatic combat circumstances among civilians when modern warfare occurs in highly populated urban zones. Thus, military and civilian casualties in modern wars engenders additional challenges to the military operational medicine, combat casualty care and the Force Health Protection healthcare program during pre-deployment, deployment and rehabilitation. These new problems demand new solutions based on advanced concepts and methods of the biosciences and health sciences, including the epidemiology of combat-related disorders. It is worth noting that the progress in understanding changes in the human body as well as in human mental ability caused by various forms of injury, including psychological trauma, can result in improved treatment of a wide variety of human diseases. Thus, these new developments can be addressed to the benefit of humanity throughout the world.

Nikolai V. Gorbunov
Henry M. Jackson Foundation for the Advancement of Military Medicine,
United States of America

Chapter 1

Introductory Chapter: Military Medicine - Current Topics

Nikolai V. Gorbunov

1. Introduction

1.1 Military medicine at the 21st century – Mission and challenges

Military medicine in the 21st Century encompasses diverse medical and scientific knowledge, techniques and combat skills to serve national military forces by optimal care of their combatants in operations on land, sea and aerospace while acting in compliance with the National Defense Strategies and International Law [1–5].

In the US Forces this also incorporates efforts on promoting health and well-being within servicemen and servicewomen that is carried out by the force health protection system [6]. Thus, along with managing illnesses and providing robust combat casualty care toward restoration of physical and mental wellness, the US military healthcare has a major stand in maintaining the readiness of members of the armed services to their missions. This burden comprises prevention of disease, injury and advancement of training and management of stress and high allostatic load in order to sustain the strength, resilience and capabilities of the personnel before, during, and after deployment [6–10].

In conjunction, it ought to be noted that there are recent growing healthcare concerns regarding environmental challenges, which are warfighters facing with in the modern operation theaters. That, along with environmental extremes and stressors (e.g., high altitude hypoxia, cold), includes emerging unconventional, asymmetric, and hybrid warfare [10, 11]. Thus, the armed conflicts or acts of terror sparking in highly populated areas, especially in urban zones, inevitably lead to devastating effects on the bystander civilian inhabitants regardless their age and sex as well as to impacts on the combatants [11–13]. In this light, increasing demand for quality of the public health and growing military needs to perform in hi-tech and stressful environments sustain endeavor to comprehend, mitigate and cure the combat-related injury and illnesses in military and civilian populations. This concept has been deliberated in current doctrines and guidelines on operational medicine and care of combat casualty of military and civilians [14]. In particular the focus of this effort is on increasing performance of far-forward surgical care with implementation of guidelines on the Pediatric Tactical Combat Casualty Care as well as on effectiveness of intensive care system [11, 15].

1.2 The burden of the combat stress-related injury and management of PTSD

It is worth emphasizing that there is high recent attention to the advancements for the long-term care of servicemen as well as to the policies on their returning to duty [3, 6–8, 14]. Thus, recent recognition of the stress-related mental illnesses as a great concern of force health protection led to development of a new concept of the US military health system that has acknowledged complicity of the injuries originated from the combat and operational stress and regarded them in the Stress Continuum Model. Note that this model adopted by the US Air Force, Army, Marine Corps and Navy has become a foundation for Combat and Operational Stress Control (COSC) and Combat Operation Control (COC) paradigm, promoting resilience, surveillance/monitoring, interventions, and management of life-altering stress problems especially, post-traumatic stress disorder (PTSD) [8, 14, 16].

PTSD has emerged as a serious mental health issue among military personal due to a broad scope of etiological factors, protracted psychological sequelae and growing socio-economical impacts of the illness; e.g., long-term medical care and life disability [14]. Evidently the combat-related PTSD in service members is more complex than in other populations. Specifically, this PTSD conditions are frequently complicated by one or more of the most common co-morbid conditions including traumatic brain injury, chronic pain and other stress disorders; and they are more difficult to treat. Moreover, often the burden of PTSD is inflamed by the negative social stigma attached to the related psychological disorders [8].

Complexity of the biological ground of the PTSD psychopathology creates significant obstacles for effective diagnostics of the disease and assessment of the alleviating treatments in the personalized therapy. In this regards, development and implementation of new techniques would be a worthwhile approach to diversify monitoring of PTSD patients [14]. This effort could also provide military psychiatrist with tools and ability to distinguish servicemen and servicewomen seeking a medical separation from active duty and some compensation through a military medical disability.

1.3 Conclusion

Over all, the analysis of the recently reported clinical studies has suggested that combat-related PTSD can be effectively treated in active duty service members. However, there are still serious challenges for the healthcare specialists in the PTSD diagnostics and management especially, in early trauma events at the far-forward combat locations.

These and other current topics of military medicine are subjects of discussion in chapters of this book.

Author details

Nikolai V. Gorbunov
Henry M. Jackson Foundation for the Advancement of Military Medicine, Bethesda, MD, United States of America

*Address all correspondence to: gorbunov.nikolaiv@gmail.com

References

[1] Casualty Care. Army Techniques Publication. No. 4-02.5. Headquarters Department of the Army. Washington, DC, 10 May 2013. https://armypubs.us.army.mil/doctrine/index.html

[2] Current Tactical Combat Casualty Care (TCCC) Guidelines 2020. Defense Health Agency. The Joint Trauma System. Committee on Tactical Combat Casualty Care. Deployed Medicine 2021. https://deployedmedicine.com/content/40

[3] Brent T. The Future of Combat Casualty Care: Is the Military Health System Ready? Santa Monica, CA: RAND Corporation, 2021. DOI:10.7249/RB-A713-1. https://www.rand.org/pubs/research_briefs/RBA713-1.html

[4] Legal Support to Military Operations. Joint Publication 1-04 (JP 1-04). US Department of Defense. 2016. https://www.jcs.mil/Portals/36/Documents/Doctrine/pubs/jp1_04.pdf

[5] Department of Defense Law of War Manual. US Department of Defense, Office of General Counsel. Washington, DC: DoD; June 2015 (Updated December 2016): Section 1.8.1.

[6] Force Health Protection. In: Army Techniques Publication 4-02.8. Headquarters, Department of the Army Washington, DC, 9 March 2016. https://armypubs.army.mil/epubs/DR_pubs/DR_a/pdf/web/atp4_02x8.pdf

[7] Riddle MS, Sanders JW, Smoak B. Force Health Protection: Prevention Deployment-Related Diseases and Non Battle Injuries. In: Out of the Crucible: How the US Military Transformed Combat Casualty Care in Iraq and Afghanistan (Textbooks of Military Medicine). Ch. 7. Eds. Kellermann AL, Elster E., U.S. Army Medical Department, The Borden Institute. US Army Medical Department Center and School Health Readiness Center of Excellence Fort Sam Houston, Texas 2017. https://bookstore.gpo.gov/products/out-crucible-how-us-military-transformed-combat-casualty-care-iraq-and-afghanistan

[8] Combat and Operational Stress Control. In: the MCCDC Doctrine. 2016 PCN 147 000045 00; NSN 0411LP110716 https://www.marines.mil/Portals/1/Publications/MCTP%20 3-30E%20Formerly%20MCRP%20 6-11C.pdf

[9] Operator Syndrome: Managing High Allostatic Load. Military.com Network. https://www.military.com/military-fitness/operator-syndrome-managing-high-allostatic-load

[10] Environmental Considerations. In: Field Manual No. 3-34.5/MCRP 4-11B (3-100.4). HEADQUARTERS, DEPARTMENT OF THE ARMY; Washington, DC. 16 February 2010 https://www.marines.mil/Portals/1/Publications/MCRP%204-11B%20 Enviromental%20Considerations.pdf?ver=2016-09-08-171729-470

[11] Kotwal RS, Staudt AM, Mazuchowski EL, Gurney JM, Shackelford SA, Butler FK, Stockinger ZT, Holcomb JB, Nessen SC, Mann-Salinas EA. A US military Role 2 forward surgical team database study of combat mortality in Afghanistan. J Trauma Acute Care Surg. 2018 Sep;85(3):603-612. doi: 10.1097/TA.0000000000001997. PMID: 29851907.

[12] Epps VC. Civilian Casualties in Modern Warfare: The Death of the Collateral Damage Rule. Ga. J. Int'l & Comp.41, 307-355 2013. https://digitalcommons.law.uga.edu/gjicl/vol41/iss2/2

[13] Annual Report on Civilian Casualties in Connection With United States

Military Operations. US Department of Defense. 2018 https://media.defense.gov/2019/May/02/2002126767/-1/-1/1/ANNUAL-REPORT-CIVILIAN-CASUALTIES-IN-CONNECTION-WITH-US-MILITARY-OPERATIONS.PDF

[14] Stewart W, Trujillo KT. Modern Warfare Destroys Brains: Creating Awareness and Educating the Force on the Effects of Blast Traumatic Brain Injury. Belfer Center for Science and International Affairs. Harvard Kennedy School. Cambridge, MA 02138 https://www.belfercenter.org/sites/default/files/2020-07/ModernWarfareDestroysBrains.pdf

[15] Pediatric Tactical Emergency Casualty Care http://www.c-tecc.org/images/content/FINAL_V.1.0_Pediatric_Guidelines.pdf

[16] Frueh BC, Madan A, Fowler JC, Stomberg S, Bradshaw M, Kelly K, Weinstein B, Luttrell M, Danner SG, Beidel DC. "Operator syndrome": A unique constellation of medical and behavioral health-care needs of military special operation forces. Int J Psychiatry Med. 2020 Jul;55(4):281-295. doi: 10.1177/0091217420906659. Epub 2020 Feb 13. PMID: 32052666.

Chapter 2

Assessment and Treatment of Combat-Related Posttraumatic Stress Disorder: Results from STRONG STAR and the Consortium to Alleviate PTSD

Alan L. Peterson, Barbara L. Niles,
Stacey Young-McCaughan and Terence M. Keane

Abstract

Extensive research has been conducted since 11 September 2001 to develop and evaluate evidence-based treatments for combat-related posttraumatic stress disorder (PTSD) in active duty United States military personnel treated in the combat theater and in garrison. This chapter reviews the results of 20 PTSD clinical trials funded by the United States Department of Defense and Department of Veterans Affairs on the treatment of combat-related PTSD. All of the studies were conducted under the leadership and management of two research consortia: the South Texas Research Organizational Network Guiding Studies on Trauma and Resilience (STRONG STAR) Consortium and the Consortium to Alleviate PTSD.

Keywords: posttraumatic stress disorder, PTSD, acute stress disorder, combat and operational stress reactions

1. Introduction

Posttraumatic stress disorder (PTSD) is a common psychiatric disorder that occurs in about 7% of the adult population after exposure to a significant traumatic event [1, 2]. Combat-related PTSD occurs as a result of exposure to military combat or other traumas experienced during military deployments. The rate of combat-related PTSD in active duty military personnel and veterans who have deployed to a combat theater of operations is about double the rate of PTSD seen in civilians. [3–6]. Prior to the terrorist attacks on the United States on September 11, 2001, most research on PTSD had been conducted with civilian and veteran populations, with a striking absence of clinical trials conducted in active duty military populations with combat-related PTSD. The need for such studies was acute because, although there are many similarities in the assessment and treatment of PTSD in civilian, veteran, and military samples, active duty personnel represent a distinct population with specific characteristics and needs. In the early- and mid-2000s, it was unclear whether methods and treatments developed for civilians would successfully translate to military personnel returning from warzones.

Combat-related PTSD in service members differs from PTSD in other populations. As compared to most civilian populations [7–9], considerable research suggests that combat-related PTSD in service members and veterans is more difficult to treat and results in a smaller percentage of patients achieving significant reductions in symptoms [10–13]. In addition, the types of traumatic events experienced in warzones are often different than for civilians [14–16] and the frequency, intensity, and duration of trauma exposure are often greater.

There are also several factors that distinguish PTSD in active duty military populations from PTSD in veteran populations and that may affect treatment and assessment. Veterans have completed their military service, are not at risk for additional combat deployments, and may receive disability compensation for their PTSD symptoms and diagnoses. Active duty military personnel with PTSD who wish to continue their military careers are faced with unique obstacles and challenges. Many service members actively avoid seeking treatment for PTSD because of the negative stigma associated with mental health treatment and concerns that a PTSD diagnosis might affect career advancement and lead to a premature discharge. Notably, U.S. military personnel who complete a minimum of 20 years of active duty service are eligible to retire at a relatively young age with a sizeable lifelong retirement pension that is often more than half of their active duty base pay in addition to other retirement benefits such a lifetime medical coverage. With few exceptions, military personnel who serve less than 20 years active service receive no military pension or benefits. As a result, there is a strong desire and incentive for many military personnel to serve on active duty for at least 20 years to be eligible for full military retirement benefits, and many are reluctant to seek care that may jeopardize this.

Assessment of PTSD relies on accurate report of symptoms, and the particular circumstances of active duty service members who do seek out treatment may impact how symptoms are reported. Many on active duty have a strong desire to be treated into remission so they can remain fully fit to continue their military service. However, there are undoubtedly some service members who actively seek a diagnosis of PTSD that will lead to separation from active duty and some compensation through a military medical disability. Despite considerable clinical and research efforts, the ability to distinguish between service members seeking continued active duty service versus those who seek a medical separation has remained difficult, and the current method is to simply ask service members their career intentions. In either instance, the service member's future career objective is challenging, but critical for the clinician to assess.

To address the lack of research on combat-related PTSD in active duty military personnel, the U.S. Congress allocated funding to Department of Defense (DoD) in 2007 through the Congressionally Directed Medical Research Programs to establish a Multidisciplinary PTSD Research Consortium. After a competitive peer-reviewed process, the STRONG STAR (South Texas Research Organizational Network Guiding Studies on Trauma And Resilience) Consortium was awarded DoD research funding in 2008 to establish a nationwide PTSD research consortium. STRONG STAR is a multidisciplinary and multi-institutional research consortium focused on the detection, diagnosis, prevention, and treatment of combat PTSD and related conditions (e.g., traumatic brain injury, sleep disorders, chronic pain, substance use disorders, suicide, etc.) in active-duty military personnel and veterans, www.STRONGSTAR.org.

The initial STRONG STAR funding supported 14 research projects and 4 research cores. STRONG STAR investigators subsequently secured additional investigator-initiated, peer-reviewed research funding through the DoD, the Department of Veterans Affairs (VA), the National Institutes of Health, and private organizations to support over 40 additional STRONG STAR-affiliated projects. In 2013, STRONG STAR investigators partnered with the VA's National Center for PTSD and were selected for joint funding by the DoD and VA to establish the Consortium to Alleviate PTSD (CAP). The CAP extended the STRONG STAR Consortium with 11 additional research projects: www.ConsortiumToAlleviatePTSD.org.

This chapter first reviews the assessment measures used to assess PTSD in the STRONG STAR and CAP studies. Next, the results of 20 STRONG STAR and CAP PTSD clinical trials evaluating a variety of treatments for combat-related PTSD in active duty military personnel and veterans are summarized.

2. The assessment of PTSD in military populations

2.1 Clinician-Administered PTSD Scale for *DSM-5*

The Clinician-Administered PTSD Scale for *DSM-5* (CAPS-5) [17, 18] is the gold-standard structured clinical diagnostic interview for assessing PTSD. The CAPS-5 is a 30-item structured clinical interview designed to be administered by a trained clinical interviewer and requires about 45–60 minutes to administer. Administration of the CAPS-5 requires the initial identification of a *DSM-5* Criterion A index traumatic event. It uses a 5-point ordinal rating scale to assess symptom the severity of the 20 PTSD symptoms included in the *DSM-5*. The CAPS-5 score can range from 0–80 with higher scores representing greater symptom severity. However, a diagnosis of PTSD is made only if the individual is experiencing ≥1 intrusion, ≥1 avoidance, ≥2 negative cognitions and mood, and ≥ 2 arousal and reactivity symptom all at a severity rating of ≥2. The CAPS-5 has strong inter-rater reliability (N = 78; *Cohen's kappa* = .90), and the correlation of severity scores between raters is excellent (r = .98) [19].

2.2 PTSD Checklist for *DSM-5*

The PTSD Checklist for *DSM-5* (PCL-5) [20] is a self-report measure of the 20 PTSD symptoms included in the *DSM-5*. Similar to the CAPS-5, it uses a 5-point ordinal rating scale to measure symptom severity with a range from 0–80. The PCL-5 can be scored in several ways, and interpretation should be made by a clinician. Initial research suggests that total scores between 31 and 33 on the PCL-5 are indicative of probable PTSD. A provisional diagnosis of PTSD can be made by summing each of the five *DSM-5* symptoms clusters with items endorsed as a 2 (Moderately) or higher and then following the *DSM-5* diagnostic guidelines. The PCL-5 has excellent psychometric characteristics for screening and as a secondary indicator of PTSD symptom severity [21, 22].

2.3 Primary Care PTSD Screen for *DSM-5*

The Primary Care PTSD Screen for *DSM-5* (PC-PTSD-5) [23] is a 5-item measure to screen for PTSD symptoms and was designed to be administered in primary care settings. The measure begins with one item to evaluate previous exposure to a potentially traumatic event. It then includes five additional yes-no items related to key PTSD symptoms. Validation studies suggest that a cut-off point of 3 on the PC-PTSD-5 is optimally sensitive for probable PTSD. Individuals who screen positive should be further evaluated with the PCL-5 or CAPS-5.

2.4 Assessment of trauma types in military personnel

Due to the unique aspects of combat- or deployment-related PTSD, the STRONG STAR investigators developed a scheme for categorizing traumatic military events [14–16]. The categorization of Criterion-A event descriptions is completed by CAPS-5 trained diagnostic interviewers. The traumatic military events are then categorized into six types of military-related Criterion-A events including (1) life-threat to self, (2) life-threat to others, (3) traumatic loss, (4) exposure to the aftermath of violence, (5) moral injury by self, and (6) moral injury by others. Research is ongoing to determine if different military trauma types respond differently to evidence-based treatments for combat-related PTSD.

2.5 The use of common data elements for PTSD research

A recent development to standardize the assessment and outcome measures that are used in PTSD research is to administer what are called *Common Data Elements*, or *CDEs* [24]. When different measures are used across studies, it makes it difficult to interpret the findings. The use of CDEs helps allow for the comparison of findings across different research studies. A major benefit of research studies conducted as part of the STRONG STAR Consortium and the Consortium to Alleviate PTSD is the use of CDEs for PTSD research [19]. This strategy also increases the possible use of future metanalytic strategies to understand the impact of various psychotherapeutic approaches in the treatment of PTSD.

3. The treatment of combat-related PTSD in military populations

At the time of the initial funding of the STRONG STAR Consortium by the DoD in 2008, no clinical trials existed to evaluate any form of treatment for combat-related PTSD in active duty military forces. Precious few randomized trials for PTSD treatment in veterans were in the published scientific literature. As a result, STRONG STAR investigators evaluated the published literature on the treatment of PTSD in civilian and veteran populations to help guide the initial studies of combat-related PTSD in active duty military personnel. The 2008 publication by the Institute of Medicine [3] titled the *Treatment of Posttraumatic Stress Disorder: An Assessment of the Evidence* provided an excellent state-of-the science review of the research literature at the time. That IOM committee report reviewed 52 psychotherapy studies and 37 pharmacotherapy studies and concluded, *"The committee finds that the evidence is sufficient to conclude the efficacy of exposure therapies in the treatment of PTSD"* [3].

Two cognitive-behavioral treatments were highlighted as the treatments with the strongest scientific support for their efficacy—Prolonged Exposure (PE) [25, 26] and Cognitive Processing Therapy (CPT) [27–29]. As a result, PE and CPT were the two treatments identified as leading candidates to be evaluated in randomized clinical trials in active duty military populations with combat-related PTSD.

Prolonged Exposure [30, 31] is a cognitive-behavioral therapy that includes four primary components: (1) imaginal exposure, or the repeated revisiting of the trauma memories, (2) in vivo exposure, or repeated exposure to avoided situations, (3) psychoeducation about common reactions to trauma, and (4) relaxed breathing. The standard treatment program includes 10 to 12 individual treatment sessions of 90 minutes each conducted once or twice a week.

Cognitive Processing Therapy is another cognitive-behavioral therapy that is usually delivered in 12 treatment sessions over the course of 6 weeks, with each session lasting 1 hour [32]. CPT begins with psychoeducation about PTSD symptoms and making connections between events, thoughts, and feelings. Patients write an "impact statement" in which they describe why they think the traumatic event happened and how the event has affected their view of themselves, others, and the world. Throughout CPT, unhelpful cognitions are identified and challenged through Socratic questioning until more helpful and accurate beliefs can replace distorted cognitions. The final five sessions of CPT focus on cognitions related to safety, trust, power, esteem, and intimacy.

A summary of the STRONG STAR and CAP clinical trials is provided in **Table 1**.

3.1 Treating combat-related PTSD in the combat theater

The first clinical case series to report on the treatment of combat-related PTSD in the combat theater [33, 34] used a modified version of Prolonged Exposure [25] that was adapted for the deployed environment. The results showed that PE could be safely and effectively delivered in the deployed environment to allow service members to return to combat duties and complete their deployments. The promising results from this case series led to the funding of a larger nonrandomized clinical trial as part of the STRONG STAR Consortium to evaluate the use of PE and CPT in Iraq and Afghanistan for the treatment of 12 service members with combat-related PTSD [35]. All patients were treated by military behavioral health providers deployed to the combat theater using modified versions of PE (n = 6) or CPT (n = 6). Because this study was conducted prior to the publication of the PCL-5, the PTSD Checklist-Military Version (PCL-M) was used [36, 37], which was based on *DSM-IV* criteria and asks about symptoms in response to "stressful military experiences." The results showed that both treatments demonstrated clinically significant change in PTSD symptoms on the PCL-M.

Despite the small sample size (N = 12), this prospective, nonrandomized trial is the largest study to date to evaluate the treatment of combat-related PTSD in the deployed combat theater. Previous military operational guidelines limited the use of trauma-focused treatments such as PE and CPT and recommended not treating PTSD until military service members returned from their deployments [38]. These recent findings should be considered in future military guidelines on the treatment of combat operational stress reactions and combat-related PTSD in the military combat theater.

3.2 Treating combat-related PTSD in military personnel in garrison

3.2.1 Prolonged Exposure Therapy

The first study to evaluate the efficacy of PE for the treatment of combat-related PTSD in active duty military personnel treated in garrison (i.e., at their non-deployed, home duty location) included 366 active duty US Army soldiers treated at Fort Hood, in Killeen, Texas. The study [39] was a 4-armed RCT to evaluate: (1) the standard delivery format of PE, which was referred to as Spaced PE (n = 109; 10 weekly 90-minute PE sessions); (2) a non-trauma focused active comparison condition called Present Centered Therapy (PCT; n = 107; 10 weekly 90-minute PCT sessions); (3) a compressed, daily format of PE called Massed PE (n = 110; 10 daily 90-minute PE sessions over 2 weeks); and a minimal-contact control condition (n = 40) involving brief, weekly phone calls from therapists to be used as a comparison condition for the Massed PE arm. The results demonstrated significant reductions in PTSD symptoms in all three active treatment arms. The Massed PE format had equivalent efficacy as the Spaced PE arm, although there were fewer dropouts

Principal Investigator/ DoD Award Number	Project Title	Interventions	Project Description	Research Participants
Jeffrey Cigrang W81XWH-08-02-0109	Brief Cognitive-Behavioral Treatment of Combat-Related PTSD in Primary Care Settings: A Pilot Study	Prolonged Exposure for Primary Care	Nonrandomized pilot clinical trial of brief cognitive-behavioral therapy (CBT) for PTSD in primary care	N = 24 Active Duty Military
Jeffrey Cigrang W81XWH-08-02-0109	Brief Cognitive-Behavioral Treatment of Combat-Related PTSD in Primary Care Settings: A Randomized Controlled Trial	Prolonged Exposure for Primary Care	RCT of brief cognitive-behavioral therapy for PTSD in primary care vs. wait list	N = 67 Active Duty Military
Edna Foa W81XWH-08-02-0111	Prolonged Exposure for PTSD in OIF/OEF Personnel: Massed versus Spaced Trials	Prolonged Exposure; Present-Centered Therapy	Four-armed RCT of spaced (weekly) PE, massed (daily) PE, present-centered therapy (PCT), or a minimal-contact control condition	N = 366 Active Duty Military
Edna Foa W81XWH-15-1-0555	60- Versus 90-Minute Prolonged Exposure for PTSD: A Randomized Control Trial in Active Duty Military Personnel	Prolonged Exposure	Two-armed RCT noninferiority trial	N = 140 Active Duty Military
Peter Fox W81XWH-13-2-0065	Image-guided, Robotically Delivered TMS for PTSD	Transcranial Magnetic Stimulation	Double-blind RCT of image-guided, robotically delivered transcranial magnetic stimulation versus sham	N = 119 (n = 114 Active Duty Military; n = 5 Veterans)
Steffany Fredman W81XWH-13-2-0065	Multi-Couple Group Intervention for PTSD	Cognitive-Behavioral Conjoint Therapy	Non-randomized clinical trial of abbreviated, intensive, multi-couple group Cognitive Behavioral Conjoint Therapy for PTSD	N = 24 Couples (n = 17 Active Duty Military; n = 7 Veterans

Principal Investigator/ DoD Award Number	Project Title	Interventions	Project Description	Research Participants
John Krystal W81XWH-13-2-0065	Ketamine for Antidepressant-Resistant PTSD	Ketamine	RCT of 0.2 mg/kg ketamine, 0.5 mg/kg ketamine, or saline placebo delivered twice per week for 4 weeks	*N* = 156 (*n* = 54 Active Duty Military; *n* = 102 Veterans)
Brian Marx W81XWH-16-2-0003	Decreasing Suicide Risk among Service Members with Posttraumatic Stress Using Written Exposure Therapy	Written Exposure Therapy for Suicide	Recruitment in Progress	Recruitment target *N* = 140 Active Duty Military
Donald McGeary W81XWH-13-2-0065	RCT of Cognitive Behavioral Therapy for PTS and Headache	Cognitive Behavior Therapy for Headache Cognitive Processing Therapy	RCT of CBT for headaches, CPT, Treatment as Usual	*N* = 193 (*n* = 3 Active Duty Military; *n* = 69 Veterans)
Carmen McLean W81XWH-14-1-0008	A Randomized Clinical Trial of Internet-Delivered PE for PTSD	Prolonged Exposure; Present-Centered Therapy	Two-armed RCT of Web-PE versus PCT	*N* = 40 (37 Active Duty Military; 3 Veterans)
Carmen McLean W81XWH-14-1-0008	A Nonrandomized Trial of Internet-Delivered PE for PTSD	Prolonged Exposure	Open clinical trial of Web-PE	*N* = 34 (2 Active Duty Military; 32 Veterans)
Candice Monson W81XWH-08-02-0115	Individual Prolonged Exposure versus Couples' Cognitive-Behavioral Therapy for Combat-Related PTSD	Cognitive Behavioral Conjoint Therapy; Prolonged Exposure	Two-armed RCT of Cognitive Behavioral Conjoint Therapy versus PE	*N* = 116 (58 Active Duty Military; 58 Military Spouses)
Alan Peterson W81XWH-08-02-0109	Outcomes of PE and CPT for Combat Operational Stress Reactions in Deployed Settings	Prolonged Exposure; Cognitive Processing Therapy	Nonrandomized clinical trial of PE and CPT delivered during a military deployment	*N* = 12 Active Duty Military
Alan Peterson W81XWH-12-2-0073	Clinical Effectiveness Trial of In-Home CPT for Combat-Related PTSD	Cognitive Processing Therapy	Three-armed RCT of In-Office, Telebehavioral Health, and In-Home CPT	*N* = 120 (*n* = 24 Active Duty Military; *n* = 96 Veterans

Principal Investigator/ DoD Award Number	Project Title	Interventions	Project Description	Research Participants
Alan Peterson W81XWH-13-2-0065	Project Remission: Maximizing Outcomes with Intensive PTSD Treatment	Prolonged Exposure	RCT of 15 daily Massed-PE or Intensive Outpatient Program-PE sessions over 3 weeks	$N = 234$ ($n = 145$ Active Duty Military; $n = 144$ Veterans)
Patricia Resick W81XWH-08-02-0116	Group Cognitive Processing Therapy versus Group Present Centered Therapy for Combat-Related PTSD	Cognitive Processing Therapy; Present-Centered Therapy	Two-armed RCT of group CPT versus group PCT	$N = 108$ Active Duty Military
Patricia Resick W81XWH-08-02-0116	Individual versus Group Cognitive Processing Therapy for Combat-Related PTSD	Cognitive Processing Therapy	Two-armed RCT of individually delivered CPT versus group-delivered CPT	$N = 268$ Active Duty Military
Patricia Resick W81XWH-13-02-0012 Alan Peterson W81XWH-13-02-0013	Variable-Length CPT for Combat-Related PTSD	Cognitive Processing Therapy	Non-randomized clinical trial of variable-lengths of CPT	$N = 130$
Denise Sloan W81XWH-15-1-0391	Brief Treatment for PTSD: Enhancing Treatment Engagement and Retention	Written Exposure Therapy	Two-armed RCT comparing WET versus CPT	$N = 170$ Active Duty Military
Daniel Taylor W81XWH-13-2-0065	Treatment of Comorbid Sleep Disorders and PTSD	Cognitive Processing Therapy; Cognitive-Behavioral Therapy for Insomnia	RCT of CPT, CPT followed by CBT-I, or CBT-I followed by CPT	$N = 94$ ($n = 87$ Active Duty Military; $n = 7$ Veterans)

Notes: CBTi = Cognitive-Behavioral Therapy for Insomnia; CPT = Cognitive Processing Therapy; CAP = Consortium to Alleviate PTSD; DoD = Department of Defense; PTSD = posttraumatic stress disorder; PCT = Present-Centered Therapy; PE = Prolonged Exposure; RCT = randomized clinical trial; STRONG STAR = South Texas Research Organizational Network Guiding Studies on Trauma and Resilience; WET = Written Exposure Therapy.

Table 1.
Summary of STRONG STAR and CAP PTSD clinical trials.

from treatment with the Massed PE format (13.6%) as compared to the Spaced PE format (24.8%), and there were fewer adverse events with the Massed PE format (25.3%) as compared to the Spaced PE format (54.1%). These results provide strong support for the compressed, Massed PE treatment format for active duty military personnel; with close coordination with military leadership, it is much easier to schedule and complete a full dose of treatment over a 2-week period as compared to weekly treatment formats that often require 3–4 months to complete.

The promising findings from the Massed PE arm of the study by Foa, McLean, and colleagues [39] led to the funding of a Consortium to Alleviate PTSD (CAP) project to further enhance the Massed PE treatment and to compare it to an Intensive Outpatient Program based on PE (IOP PE). The CAP study [40] randomized 234 active duty service members and veterans to either 15 sessions of daily Massed PE or IOP PE treatment over a 3-week period. The IOP PE arm included eight enhancements to the Massed PE protocol that targeted many of the unique aspects of combat-related PTSD. The enhancements included (1) a team-based treatment approach, rather than relying on one therapist; (2) completion of daily homework assignments at the clinic; (3) 15- to 30-minute, in-person feedback sessions after daily homework assignments; (4) active involvement of the spouse or other support person for in vivo exposures; (5) targeting the patients' top three most distressing traumas during imaginal exposure; (6) starting imaginal exposure with the least distressing trauma and progressing to the most distressing trauma; (7) a brief review of all other potentially traumatic events that occurred during previous deployments; and (8) the completion of three posttreatment booster sessions. The final results of this study have not yet been published, but preliminary results [41] indicate that both treatments resulted in large reductions in PTSD symptoms at the conclusion of treatment, but only those randomized to the IOP PE maintained the large treatment gains over the 6-month follow-up period. The reduction of PTSD symptoms and maintenance of treatment gains with the IOP PE arm are among the strongest treatment outcomes to date for combat-related PTSD.

Another adaptation of the standard, weekly, 90-minute outpatient format for PE was a series of STRONG STAR studies designed to adapt PE for use in military primary care clinics. The first project was a pilot study ($N = 24$) to develop and test an abbreviated PE protocol adapted for primary care (called PE for Primary Care) consisting of four to six 30-minute treatment sessions conducted by a behavioral health consultant embedded in an integrated primary care clinic. The results showed that PTSD severity was significantly reduced and 50% of the patients no longer met criteria for PTSD after treatment [42, 43].

The results of the pilot project were then used in a subsequent RCT in which 67 service members were randomized to receive the PE for Primary Care treatment or a minimal contact control condition followed by treatment after 6 weeks [44]. The results indicated that the immediate treatment group had large reductions in PTSD severity as compared to the minimal contact control. Similar improvements were found in the delayed treatment group when they received the PE for Primary Care treatment, and the treatment benefits persisted through the 6-month follow-up point for all participants. These finding suggest that an abbreviated version of PE delivered in integrated primary care clinics is effective for the treatment of PTSD and may help reduce barriers and stigma found in specialty care settings.

Another adaptation of the standard outpatient PE protocol was the development of a web-based version of PE [45] to help improve accessibility of effective and efficient evidence-based treatments for PTSD. Web-PE was first compared to in-person Present-Centered Therapy in an RCT with 40 military personnel with PTSD at Fort Hood, Texas. Due to recruitment challenges in the RCT, the efficacy of the Web-PE treatment was then evaluated in an open trial with 34 service members and veterans recruited nationwide. The results of the RCT showed that both Web-PE and PCT significantly reduced interviewer-assessed and self-reported symptoms of PTSD, with no significant differences between the groups and a medium effect size for Web-PE [46]. The open trial of Web-PE showed significant reductions in self-reported PTSD symptoms with a large effect size. These results suggest that Web-PE is a potential alternative to standard, in-person PE, although the benefits in reducing PTSD symptoms are likely to be greater in patients who are specifically seeking a web-based treatment.

A significant limitation of the outpatient version of PE for the treatment of military personnel in garrison is that delivering the standard 90-minute PE sessions is difficult in many military mental health settings. To address this challenge, an RCT was conducted to evaluate the efficacy of 60-minute versus 90-minute PE sessions [47]. The preliminary results indicate that the shorter sessions possess equal efficacy, thereby increasing the potential feasibility of using the 60-minute format in military mental health settings [48].

3.2.2 Cognitive Processing Therapy

The first study to evaluate the efficacy of CPT for the treatment of combat-related PTSD in active duty military personnel treated in garrison included 108 active duty US Army soldiers treated at Fort Hood, in Killeen, Texas [49]. The study was an RCT to compare group CPT to group Present-Centered Therapy (PCT). Participants were randomized to attend twice weekly 90-minute group treatments of CPT or PCT. The results indicated that both treatments resulted in large reductions in both clinician-administered and self-report measures of PTSD symptoms, but the group CPT treatment resulted in larger reductions [49].

As a follow-on study to the group CPT versus group PCT, another RCT ($N = 268$) was conducted at Fort Hood to compare CPT delivered in a group format to CPT delivered in an individual format [50]. The study was designed as a noninferiority trial and hypothesized that group CPT would function as well as individual CPT in reducing symptoms. If proved true, group CPT would be more efficient to deliver to a larger proportion of active duty military patients with the need for fewer therapists. The results, however, did not support this hypothesis. Individual CPT was found to be significantly more effective in reducing PTSD symptoms compared to group CPT. The findings suggest that the effective treatment of PTSD with CPT requires a focus on the specific traumas and related cognitions that are unique to individual patients. However, even among those receiving individual CPT, approximately one-half still had clinically significant PTSD symptoms, indicating that additional improvements are needed for existing treatments.

To address these concerns, a study was conducted modeled after a study conducted with civilians that demonstrated treatment outcomes could be improved by varying the number of CPT sessions based on patient response to treatment. The study was conducted using a nonrandomized, within-group design treating 127 active duty military personnel [51]. Patients received variable-length CPT which could end before 12 sessions or extend up to 24 sessions over 18 weeks if patient and therapist agreed a good end state had been reached (PCL-5 $\leq$ 19). The results indicated that the variable-length CPT outcomes were superior to the previous fixed-length CPT studies conducted with military personnel in proportion to diagnostic remission on the CAPS-5 (65% vs. 40%) and clinically significant symptom improvement on the PCL-5 (76% vs. 46%) [52].

Another method to address some of the potential limitations of the standard CPT protocol is to evaluate different delivery settings for CPT. To evaluate these factors, an RCT was conducted to determine if CPT delivered face-to-face in a patient's home (In-Home CPT) or by telehealth to their home (Telehealth CPT) would result in increased acceptability, fewer dropouts, and better outcomes for service members and veterans than standard In-Office CPT [53]. This study used an equipoise stratified randomization design in which participants could opt out of one delivery modality and still be randomized to one of the other two.

The results showed that 57% of participants declined one of the treatment arms (In-Home = 30%; In-Office = 16%; Telehealth = 11%). However, dropout from treatment was lowest when therapy was delivered In-Home (21%) as compared to Telehealth (33%) and In-Office (44%) [54]. Significant reductions in PTSD symptoms occurred across all three treatments, and a remarkable 56% of participants no longer met diagnostic criteria for PTSD at the end of treatment. Treatment outcomes were better when patients received more treatment, and improvements were considerably better when CPT was delivered In-Home or by Telehealth. An additional advantage of the Telehealth CPT is that it reduced the average patient and therapist time commitment by 50% as compared to the In-Office or In-Home treatments. CPT delivered by telehealth is also an efficient and effective treatment modality for PTSD in active duty military. This is an important scientific observation considering recent limitations to in-person care resulting from the COVID-19 pandemic.

Although CPT was designed for the treatment of PTSD related to sexual assault in civilians, there is increasing evidence that it may also be helpful for PTSD that is comorbid with other deployment-related disorders such as posttraumatic headache and insomnia. One CAP 3-armed RCT (N = 193) compared CPT, Cognitive-Behavioral Therapy for Headache, and treatment as usual for veterans and active duty service members with comorbid posttraumatic and PTSD symptoms [55]. The results indicated that, compared to treatment as usual, both CPT and Cognitive-Behavioral Therapy for Headache reduced PTSD symptoms on the PCL-5, but only Cognitive-Behavioral Therapy for Headache reduced headache disability symptoms [56].

Furthermore, one CAP study evaluated the sequencing of treatment for comorbid PTSD and insomnia [57] in military service members and veterans (N = 94). The RCT compared (1) 18 sessions of CPT alone, (2) 12 session of CPT followed by 6 sessions of Cognitive-Behavioral Therapy for Insomnia (CBT-I), or (3) 6 sessions of CBT-I followed by 12 sessions of CPT. The preliminary results [58] suggest that treatment sequencing matters and that there are greater reductions in PTSD symptoms when CPT is used first and is followed by CBT-I. Conversely, improved outcomes for insomnia occur when CBT-I is used first and followed by CPT.

3.2.3 Cognitive-Behavioral Conjoint Therapy

Cognitive-Behavioral Conjoint Therapy (CBCT) [59] is a couples-based, 15-session, weekly treatment program to address both PTSD symptoms and relationship functioning. Despite previous research to support the efficacy of CBCT in civilian and veteran couples, the first RCT with active duty military couples comparing CBCT to PE failed to replicate previous results [60]. One of the primary challenges in conducting CBCT with military couples was that the military work environment made it very difficult for both spouses to attend the proposed 15 treatment sessions, resulting in a high dropout rate. To address these challenges, the treatment protocol was redesigned as an abbreviated, intensive, multi-couple group version of CBCT in which the entire treatment protocol was delivered as a 2-day weekend retreat [61]. The results of a nonrandomized clinical trial (N = 24 couples) that included an active duty service member or veteran who had previously deployed found significant reductions in both clinician-rated and self-reported PTSD symptoms as well as significant improvements in relationship satisfaction. However, the results are limited by the nonrandomized design used for this pilot project. Additional research is needed comparing the abbreviated, intensive, multi-couple group version of CBCT to an active comparison intervention.

3.2.4 Written Exposure Therapy

One of the more recent developments to improve treatment efficacy and efficiency for PTSD and decrease dropout rates is a 5-session treatment called Written Exposure Therapy (WET) [62]. After almost 20 years of research with civilian and veteran populations to investigate imaginal exposure in a written form, the first RCT to treat service members in garrison was a 2-armed noninferiority RCT (N = 170) comparing WET to CPT [63]. The results indicated that the 5-session WET protocol was equally effective as the 12-session CPT protocol. However, dropouts from treatment were significantly less for WET (24%) as compared to CPT (45%). The results demonstrate that WET is an efficient method to treat combat-related PTSD and results in fewer dropouts from treatment and may well represent an important treatment improvement from a public health perspective (i.e., fewer sessions needed and fewer dropouts).

The results of this initial WET study provided support for a follow-on study to evaluate a modified version of WET targeting co-morbid PTSD symptoms and suicidal ideations (WET-S) for service members hospitalized on a military psychiatric inpatient facility. Crisis Response Planning was added to the standard WET protocol to address the suicidal ideations. Recruitment is ongoing for this study, but preliminary results appear quite promising [64].

3.2.5 Medications and devices for the treatment of PTSD in military personnel

Although exposure-based cognitive-behavioral treatments have the largest number of studies supporting the efficacy in treating PTSD, other approaches exist and are promising. One CAP study was a double-blind RCT ($N = 119$) comparing 20 sessions of image-guided, robotically delivered transcranial magnetic stimulation (irTMS) to a sham TMS in service members and veterans hospitalized in a private psychiatric facility in San Antonio, Texas [65]. The treatment for PTSD was delivered to the right dorsolateral prefrontal cortex, an area related to the neural circuitry for stress and anxiety disorders. The preliminary results indicated that there were greater PCL-5 score reductions for active irTMS than for sham at every assessment time point.

Another CAP study was the largest RCT to date to evaluate ketamine for antidepressant-resistant PTSD in 156 service members and veterans randomized to 0.2 mg/kg ketamine, 0.5 mg/kg ketamine, or saline placebo delivered twice per week for 4 weeks [66]. The preliminary results indicated that there were no statistically significant differences in reductions in PTSD among any of the treatment arms; however, there were significant reductions in depression with the higher dose of ketamine. More data analyses are ongoing to more fully understand the impact of ketamine treatment for combat-related PTSD.

4. Summary and conclusions

Over the past decade, the STRONG STAR Consortium and the Consortium to Alleviate PTSD successfully completed 20 clinical trials to evaluate various treatment interventions for combat-related PTSD in active duty military personnel. These studies documented that combat-related PTSD can be effectively treated in military personnel, with up to 80% having significant reductions in their PTSD symptoms and about one-half no longer meeting diagnostic criteria for PTSD at the end of treatment. Importantly, a clinical case series demonstrated that trauma-focused treatments to address combat operational stress reactions and combat-related PTSD can be successfully delivered in the military combat theater [33, 34]. Several studies presented above successfully adapted PE for military populations in various ways to improve access, reduce dropout, and enhance outcomes. These include shortening the time between sessions [39, 40], reducing the number of sessions [42–44], providing web-based treatment [46], reducing the length of sessions [47], and conducting intensive weekend retreats for couples [61]. Similarly, a variable length CPT protocol successfully treated active duty military with improved outcomes [51] and demonstrated efficacy in multiple in-person or telehealth settings [54]. A study showing individually delivered CPT to be more efficacious than CPT delivered in a group format [50] has important implications for health care delivery in both military and VA facilities. Studies of the treatment of comorbid posttraumatic headache [56] and insomnia [58] showed that CPT can be successfully paired with other treatments to improve outcomes. A pilot study of conjoint treatment for military couples using a weekend retreat format shows great promise for reducing PTSD symptoms as well as enhancing relationship satisfaction [59]. Finally, WET, a 5-session written exposure treatment, has been shown to treat service members in garrison as successfully as a 12-session CPT but with lower dropout [63]. Despite these important advances, there remains a critical need for research to further improve upon the assessment, diagnosis, treatment, and prevention of PTSD and comorbid conditions in service members and veterans.

Findings from multiple clinical trials have now demonstrated combat-related PTSD can be effectively treated in active duty service members and veterans, but there are additional challenges in the treatment of these populations as compared to many civilian traumas. The assessment and treatment approaches for these conditions must be adapted and tailored for the unique aspects of combat-related traumas and for PTSD that is complicated by one or more of the most common comorbid conditions including TBI, sleep disorders, substance use disorders, chronic pain, and risk for suicide. Clinical trials are also needed to further evaluate the combination of cognitive-behavioral therapies with medications and medical devices. In addition, brief interventions that can be administered soon after trauma exposure in far-forward combat locations need to be evaluated as methods to prevent the onset of chronic PTSD.

Funding

The authors' work on this chapter was supported by Consortium to Alleviate PTSD (CAP) award numbers W81XWH-13-2-0065 from the U.S. Department of Defense, Defense Health Program, Psychological Health and Traumatic Brain Injury Research Program (PH/TBI RP), and I01CX001136-01 from the U.S. Department of Veterans Affairs, Office of Research & Development, Clinical Science Research & Development Service.

Disclaimer

The views expressed herein are solely those of the authors and do not reflect an endorsement by or the official policy or position of the the Department of Defense, the Department of Veterans Affairs, or the U.S. Government.

Author details

Alan L. Peterson[1,2,3]*, Barbara L. Niles[4,5], Stacey Young-McCaughan[1,2] and Terence M. Keane[4,5]

1 University of Texas Health Science Center at San Antonio, San Antonio, Texas, USA

2 South Texas Veterans Health Care System, San Antonio, Texas, USA

3 University of Texas at San Antonio, San Antonio, Texas, USA

4 National Center for PTSD, VA Boston Healthcare System, Boston, Massachusetts, USA

5 Boston University School of Medicine, Boston, Massachusetts, USA

*Address all correspondence to: petersona3@uthscsa.edu

References

[1] Kessler RC, Aguilar-Gaxiola S, Alonso J, et al. Trauma and PTSD in the WHO World Mental Health Surveys. *Eur J Psychotraumatol*. 2017;8(sup5):1353383. Published 2017 Oct 27. doi:10.1080/20008198.2017.1353383

[2] Kilpatrick DG, Resnick HS, Milanak ME, Miller MW, Keyes KM, Friedman MJ. National estimates of exposure to traumatic events and PTSD prevalence using DSM-IV and DSM-5 criteria. *J Trauma Stress*. 2013;26(5):537-547. doi:10.1002/jts.21848

[3] Institute of Medicine. *Treatment of Posttraumatic Stress Disorder: An Assessment of the Evidence*. The National Academies Press; 2008.

[4] Institute of Medicine. *Treatment of Posttraumatic Stress Disorder in Military and Veteran Populations: Final Assessment*. The National Academies Press; 2014.

[5] Judkins JL, Moore BA, Collette TL, Hale WJ, Peterson AL, Morissette SB. Incidence Rates of Posttraumatic Stress Disorder Over a 17-Year Period in Active Duty Military Service Members. *J Trauma Stress*. 2020;33(6):994-1006. doi:10.1002/jts.22558

[6] Tanielian T, Jaycox, LH, eds. *Invisible Wounds of War: Psychological and Cognitive Injuries, Their Consequences, and Services to Assist Recovery.* RAND Corporation; 2008

[7] Bisson J, Andrew M. Psychological treatment of post-traumatic stress disorder (PTSD). *Cochrane Database Syst Rev*. 2007;(3):CD003388. Published 2007 Jul 18. doi:10.1002/14651858.CD003388.pub3.

[8] Bisson JI, Ehlers A, Matthews R, Pilling S, Richards D, Turner S. Psychological treatments for chronic post-traumatic stress disorder. Systematic review and meta-analysis. *Br J Psychiatry*. 2007;190:97-104. doi:10.1192/bjp.bp.106.021402

[9] Foa EB, Keane TM, Friedman, MJ, eds. *Effective Treatments for PTSD: Practice Guidelines from the Intrnational Society for Traumatic Stress Studies.* Guilford Publications; 2000

[10] Hoge CW, Auchterlonie JL, Milliken CS. Mental health problems, use of mental health services, and attrition from military service after returning from deployment to Iraq or Afghanistan. *JAMA*. 2006;295(9):1023-1032. doi:10.1001/jama.295.9.1023

[11] Hoge CW, Terhakopian A, Castro CA, Messer SC, Engel CC. Association of posttraumatic stress disorder with somatic symptoms, health care visits, and absenteeism among Iraq war veterans. *Am J Psychiatry*. 2007;164(1):150-153. doi:10.1176/ajp.2007.164.1.150

[12] Milliken CS, Auchterlonie JL, Hoge CW. Longitudinal assessment of mental health problems among active and reserve component soldiers returning from the Iraq war. *JAMA*. 2007;298(18):2141-2148. doi:10.1001/jama.298.18.2141

[13] Steenkamp MM, Litz BT, Hoge CW, Marmar CR. Psychotherapy for Military-Related PTSD: A Review of Randomized Clinical Trials. *JAMA*. 2015;314(5):489-500. doi:10.1001/jama.2015.8370

[14] Litz BT, Contractor AA, Rhodes C, et al. Distinct Trauma Types in Military Service Members Seeking Treatment for Posttraumatic Stress Disorder. *J Trauma Stress*. 2018;31(2):286-295. doi:10.1002/jts.22276

[15] Presseau C, Litz BT, Kline NK, et al. An epidemiological evaluation of

trauma types in a cohort of deployed service members. *Psychol Trauma*. 2019;11(8):877-885. doi:10.1037/tra0000465

[16] Stein NR, Mills MA, Arditte K, et al. A scheme for categorizing traumatic military events. *Behav Modif*. 2012;36(6):787-807. doi:10.1177/0145445512446945

[17] Weathers FW, Blake DD, Schnurr PP, et al. *The Clinician-Administered PTSD Scale for DSM-5 (CAPS-5)*. 2013. https://www.ptsd.va.gov.

[18] Weathers FW, Bovin MJ, Lee DJ, et al. The Clinician-Administered PTSD Scale for DSM-5 (CAPS-5): Development and initial psychometric evaluation in military veterans. *Psychol Assess*. 2018;30(3):383-395. doi:10.1037/pas0000486

[19] Barnes BJ, Presseau C, Jordan AH, et al. Common Data Elements in the Assessment of Military-Related PTSD Research Applied in the Consortium to Alleviate PTSD. *Mil Med*. 2019;184(5-6):e218-e226. doi:10.1093/milmed/usy226

[20] Weathers FW, Litz BT, Keane TM, et al. *The PTSD Checklist for DSM-5 (PCL-5)*. 2013. https://www.ptsd.va.gov/professional/assessment/adult-sr/ptsd-checklist.asp.

[21] Bovin MJ, Marx BP, Weathers FW, et al. Psychometric properties of the PTSD Checklist for Diagnostic and Statistical Manual of Mental Disorders-Fifth Edition (PCL-5) in veterans. *Psychol Assess*. 2016;28(11):1379-1391. doi:10.1037/pas0000254

[22] Wortmann JH, Jordan AH, Weathers FW, et al. Psychometric analysis of the PTSD Checklist-5 (PCL-5) among treatment-seeking military service members. *Psychol Assess*. 2016;28(11):1392-1403. doi:10.1037/pas0000260

[23] Prins A, Bovin MJ, Kimerling R, et al. Primary Care PTSD Screen for DSM-5 (PC-PTSD-5). 2015. https://www.ptsd.va.gov

[24] Kaloupek DG, Chard KM, Freed MC, et al. Common data elements for posttraumatic stress disorder research. *Arch Phys Med Rehabil*. 2010;91(11):1684-1691. doi:10.1016/j.apmr.2010.06.032

[25] Foa EB, Dancu CV, Hembree EA, Jaycox LH, Meadows EA, Street GP. A comparison of exposure therapy, stress inoculation training, and their combination for reducing posttraumatic stress disorder in female assault victims. *J Consult Clin Psychol*. 1999;67(2):194-200. doi:10.1037//0022-006x.67.2.194

[26] Foa EB, Hembree EA, Cahill SP, et al. Randomized trial of prolonged exposure for posttraumatic stress disorder with and without cognitive restructuring: outcome at academic and community clinics. *J Consult Clin Psychol*. 2005;73(5):953-964. doi:10.1037/0022-006X.73.5.953

[27] Monson CM, Fredman SJ, Adair KC. Cognitive-behavioral conjoint therapy for posttraumatic stress disorder: application to operation enduring and Iraqi Freedom veterans. *J Clin Psychol*. 2008;64(8):958-971. doi:10.1002/jclp.20511

[28] Resick PA, Nishith P, Weaver TL, Astin MC, Feuer CA. A comparison of cognitive-processing therapy with prolonged exposure and a waiting condition for the treatment of chronic posttraumatic stress disorder in female rape victims. *J Consult Clin Psychol*. 2002;70(4):867-879. doi:10.1037//0022-006x.70.4.867

[29] Resick PA, Galovski TE, Uhlmansiek MO, Scher CD, Clum GA,

Young-Xu Y. A randomized clinical trial to dismantle components of cognitive processing therapy for posttraumatic stress disorder in female victims of interpersonal violence. *J Consult Clin Psychol*. 2008;76(2):243-258. doi:10.1037/0022-006X.76.2.243

[30] Foa EB, Hembree EA, Rothbaum BO. *Prolonged Exposure Therapy for PTSD: Emotional Processing Of Traumatic Experiences Therapist Guide;*Oxford University Press. 2007

[31] Peterson AL, Foa EB, Riggs DS. Prolonged exposure therapy. In Moore BA, Penk W, eds. *Treating PTSD in Military Personnel: A Clinical Handbook, 2nd ed.* Guilford; 2019: 46-62

[32] Resick PA, Monson CM, Chard KM. *Cognitive Processing Therapy for PTSD: Comprehensive Manual.* Guilford Press; 2017

[33] Cigrang JA, Peterson AL, Schobitz RP. Three American troops in Iraq: Evaluation of a brief exposure therapy treatment for the secondary prevention of combat-related PTSD. *Prag Case Stud Psychother. 2005;1*(2). doi.org/10.14713/pcsp.v1i2.857

[34] Peterson AL, Cigrang JA, Schobitz RP. Response to commentaries: the scientist-practitioner on the front line: development and formalization of evidenced-based interventions on the battlefield. *Prag Case Stud Psychother.* 2005;1,(2), Article 4;1-5. doi.org/10.14713/pcsp.v1i2.859

[35] Peterson AL, Foa EB, Resick PA, et al. A Nonrandomized Trial of Prolonged Exposure and Cognitive Processing Therapy for Combat-Related Posttraumatic Stress Disorder in a Deployed Setting. *Behav Ther*. 2020;51(6):882-894. doi:10.1016/j.beth.2020.01.003

[36] Weathers FW, Litz BT, Herman DS, Huska JA, Keane TM. The PTSD Checklist (PCL): Reliability, validity, and diagnostic utility. Paper presented at the 9th annual meeting of the International Society for Traumatic Stress Studies; October 25, 1993; San Antonio, Texas.

[37] Bliese PD, Wright KM, Adler AB, Cabrera O, Castro CA, Hoge CW. Validating the primary care posttraumatic stress disorder screen and the posttraumatic stress disorder checklist with soldiers returning from combat. *J Consult Clin Psychol*. 2008;76(2):272-281. doi:10.1037/0022-006X.76.2.272

[38] Peterson AL, Straud CL, Evans WR. Treating combat-related posttraumatic stress disorder during military deployments: importance, challenges, and special considerations. *The Behav Ther.* 2019;42:127-131. http://www.abct.org/Journals/?m=mJournal&fa=TBT

[39] Foa EB, McLean CP, Zang Y, et al. Effect of Prolonged Exposure Therapy Delivered Over 2 Weeks vs 8 Weeks vs Present-Centered Therapy on PTSD Symptom Severity in Military Personnel: A Randomized Clinical Trial [published correction appears in JAMA. 2018 Aug 21;320(7):724]. *JAMA*. 2018;319(4):354-364. doi:10.1001/jama.2017.21242

[40] Peterson AL, Foa EB, Blount TH, et al. Intensive prolonged exposure therapy for combat-related posttraumatic stress disorder: Design and methodology of a randomized clinical trial. *Contemp Clin Trials*. 2018;72:126-136. doi:10.1016/j.cct.2018.07.016

[41] Peterson AL, Blount TH, Foa EB, et al. Intensive prolonged exposure for combat-related PTSD: Results from a randomized clinical trial In Keane TM (chair), The Consortium to Alleviate Posttraumatic Stress Disorder Symposium. Paper accepted for presentation at: 40th Annual Conference of the Anxiety and Depression Association of America; March 20,

2020; San Antonio, TX. (Conference cancelled)

[42] Cigrang JA, Rauch SA, Avila LL, et al. Treatment of active-duty military with PTSD in primary care: early findings. *Psych Serv.* 2011;*8*(2):104-113. doi:10.1037/a0022740.

[43] Cigrang JA, Rauch SA, Mintz J, et al. Treatment of active duty military with PTSD in primary care: A follow-up report. *J Anxiety Disord*. 2015;36:110-114. doi:10.1016/j.janxdis.2015.10.003

[44] Cigrang JA, Rauch SA, Mintz J, et al. Moving effective treatment for posttraumatic stress disorder to primary care: A randomized controlled trial with active duty military. *Fam Syst Health*. 2017;35(4):450-462. doi:10.1037/fsh0000315

[45] McLean CP, Rauch SAM, Foa EB, et al. Design of a randomized controlled trial examining the efficacy and biological mechanisms of web-prolonged exposure and present-centered therapy for PTSD among active-duty military personnel and veterans. *Contemp Clin Trials*. 2018;64:41-48. doi:10.1016/j.cct.2017.11.008

[46] McLean CP, Foa EB, Dondanville KA, et al. The effects of web-prolonged exposure among military personnel and veterans with posttraumatic stress disorder [published online ahead of print, 2020 Nov 19]. *Psychol Trauma*. 2020;10.1037/tra0000978. doi:10.1037/tra0000978

[47] Foa EB, Zandberg LJ, McLean CP, et al. The efficacy of 90-minute versus 60-minute sessions of prolonged exposure for posttraumatic stress disorder: Design of a randomized controlled trial in active duty military personnel. *Psychol Trauma*. 2019;11(3):307-313. doi:10.1037/tra0000351

[48] Foa EB. 90-minute versus 60-minute sessions of prolonged exposure for the treatment of PTSD. Paper presented at: 5th Annual San Antonio Combat PTSD Conference; October 23, 2020; San Antonio, Texas.

[49] Resick PA, Wachen JS, Mintz J, et al. A randomized clinical trial of group cognitive processing therapy compared with group present-centered therapy for PTSD among active duty military personnel. *J Consult Clin Psychol*. 2015;83(6):1058-1068. doi:10.1037/ccp0000016

[50] Resick PA, Wachen JS, Dondanville KA, et al. Effect of Group vs Individual Cognitive Processing Therapy in Active-Duty Military Seeking Treatment for Posttraumatic Stress Disorder: A Randomized Clinical Trial [published correction appears in JAMA Psychiatry. 2017 Jun 1;74(6):655]. *JAMA Psychiatry*. 2017;74(1):28-36. doi:10.1001/jamapsychiatry.2016.2729

[51] Wachen JS, Dondanville KA, Young-McCaughan S, et al. Testing a variable-length Cognitive Processing Therapy intervention for posttraumatic stress disorder in active duty military: Design and methodology of a clinical trial. *Contemp Clin Trials Commun*. 2019;15:100381. Published 2019 May 23. doi:10.1016/j.conctc.2019.100381

[52] Wachen JS, Mintz J, Dondanville KA, et al. *Variable-length cognitive processing therapy: predicting length of treatment to good end state in an active duty military sample.* Poster presented at: Annual Meeting of the International Society for Traumatic Stress Studies; November 15, 2019; Boston, MA.

[53] Peterson AL, Resick PA, Mintz J, et al. Design of a clinical effectiveness trial of in-home cognitive processing therapy for combat-related PTSD. *Contemp Clin Trials*. 2018;73:27-35. doi:10.1016/j.cct.2018.08.005

[54] Peterson AL, Mintz J, Moring J, et al. In-office, in-home, and telebehavioral-health cognitive processing therapy for combat-related PTSD: preliminary results of a randomized clinical trial. Paper presented at: 4th Annual San Antonio Combat PTSD Conference; October 24, 2019; San Antonio, TX.

[55] McGeary DD, Penzien DB, Resick PA, et al. Study design for a randomized clinical trial of cognitive-behavioral therapy for posttraumatic headache. *Contemp Clin Trials*. 2021;21. doi.org/10.1016/j.conctc.2021.100699.

[56] McGeary DD. Non-pharmacological management of posttraumatic headache in post-9/11 veterans: a Consortium to Alleviate PTSD study. In Keane TM (chair), *The Consortium to Alleviate Posttraumatic Stress Disorder Symposium*. Paper accepted for presentation at: 40th Annual Conference of the Anxiety and Depression Association of America; March 20, 2020; San Antonio, TX. (Conference cancelled)

[57] Taylor DJ, Pruiksma KE, Mintz J, et al. Treatment of comorbid sleep disorders and posttraumatic stress disorder in active duty military: Design and methodology of a randomized clinical trial. *Contemp Clin Trials*. 2020;99:106186. doi:10.1016/j.cct.2020.106186

[58] Taylor DJ, Resick PA, Pruiksma KE, et al. Treatment of comorbid sleep disorders and PTSD. Paper presented at: Annual Meeting of the International Society for Traumatic Stress Studies; November 15, 2019; Boston, MA.

[59] Monson CM, Fredman SJ. *Cognitive-behavioral conjoint therapy for posttraumatic stress disorder: harnessing the healing power of relationships.* Guilford Press; 2012

[60] Monson CM. Cognitive-behavioral conjoint therapy versus prolonged exposure for military-related PTSD: primary outcomes from a randomized controlled trial. Paper presented at: 2nd San Antonio Combat PTSD Conference; October 19, 2017; San Antonio, Texas.

[61] Fredman SJ, Macdonald A, Monson CM, et al. Intensive, Multi-Couple Group Therapy for PTSD: A Nonrandomized Pilot Study With Military and Veteran Dyads. *Behav Ther*. 2020;51(5):700-714. doi:10.1016/j.beth.2019.10.003

[62] Sloan DM Marx BP. *Written Exposure Therapy for PTSD: A Brief Treatment Approach for Mental Health Professionals*. American Psychological Association; 2019.

[63] Sloan DM, Marx BP, Resick PA, et al. Study design comparing written exposure therapy to cognitive processing therapy for PTSD among military service members: A noninferiority trial. *Contemp Clin Trials Commun*. 2019;17:100507. Published 2019 Dec 10. doi:10.1016/j.conctc.2019.100507

[64] Tyler HC, Fina BA, Marx BP, et al. (under review). Written Exposure Therapy for suicide in a psychiatric inpatient unit: a case series.

[65] Fox PT, Salinas F, Roache JD, et al. Image-guided, robotically delivered transcranial magnetic stimulation (irTMS) for combat-related PTSD: preliminary results of a randomized controlled trial. Paper presented at: 4th Annual San Antonio Combat PTSD Conference; October 24, 2019; San Antonio, Texas.

[66] Abdallah CG, Roache JD, Averill LA, et al. Repeated ketamine infusions for antidepressant-resistant PTSD: Methods of a multicenter, randomized, placebo-controlled clinical trial. *Contemp Clin Trials*. 2019;81:11-18. doi:10.1016/j.cct.2019.04.009

Chapter 3

Chemokines as Potential Biomarkers for PTSD in Military Population

Lei Zhang, Xianzhang Hu, Xiaoxia Li and Robert J. Ursano

Abstract

Post-traumatic stress disorder (PTSD) is a serious mental health concern worldwide among civilians and military personnel. Gaps in our understanding of its biological basis create significant obstacles for accurate diagnosis and assessment of therapeutic interventions. In light of this, investigation of biological factors associated with possible molecular cues of inflammation or neuroimmune disorders, could provide new surrogate markers for PTSD or PTSD treatment response. Analyses to date in deployed military personnel have suggested that sets of chemokines may be useful as biomarkers for PTSD acquired in military operations. Specifically, studies to date suggest that CCL2, CCL15, CCL22, CCL25, CXCL2, and CXCL12 are associated with PTSD onset, while CCL13, CCL20, and CXCL6 are correlated to PTSD risk; CX3CL1 are associated with resilience; CCL3; CXCL11, and CXCL16 are associated with stress response. CCL11, CCL13, CCL20, and CCL25 are correlated with the severity of PTSD symptoms. This chapter reviews the current understanding of potential chemokine markers for PTSD, and the potential chemokines associated with PTSD onset, risk, resilience, as well as stress responses in service members. Although the proposed biomarkers require further validation, these findings may lead to additional knowledge for the education and development of diagnostic and therapeutic approaches for PTSD, not only benefiting military personnel, but civilians as well.

Keywords: Post-traumatic stress disorder, PTSD, cytokine, chemokine, biomarker

1. Introduction

Post-traumatic stress disorder (PTSD) is a stress related disorder. Its lifetime prevalence in U.S. general population is about 7% to 9% and the point prevalence of PTSD in combat veterans is 17% [1]. During the Iraq and Afghanistan Wars, the point prevalence was significantly increased in the military population. About 10–18% of service members manifest probable PTSD following deployment (https://www.ptsd.va.gov/public/PTSD-overview/basics/how-common-is-ptsd.asp). The neuropsychological impairments of PTSD can be debilitating, and significantly affect mental and physical function. Cognitive-behavioral psychotherapies are used to treat patients [2–4]. There are only two US Food and Drug Administration (FDA) approved medications for PTSD, sertraline and paroxetine, which are selective serotonin reuptake inhibitor antidepressants [5]. However, their therapeutic efficacy is not sufficient in some patients. Moreover, the molecular mechanisms underlying PTSD remain largely unknown. Presently, PTSD diagnosis is based on clinical history, mental status, symptom duration, and symptom checklists or patient self-reports and lack of objective biomarker tests. To begin early intervention, objective diagnostic approaches are needed. Progress is being make [6]. Thus, a diagnostic biomarker test in the early stage or a treatable stage of the disorder would be beneficial for physicians and patients.

Biomarker research has been incrementally translated into clinical applications and has provided the necessary platform for development of novel therapeutic [7] and diagnosis approaches. One emerging area in PTSD research is the association studies regarding central nervous system (CNS)-specific immune proteins such as cytokines and chemokines. Several studies have demonstrated that cytokines play a role in brain development and function, and affect the neural circuits and transmitters within the brain, causing changes in behavior. The levels of pro-inflammatory cytokines such as interleukin (IL)-1, IL-6, tumor necrosis factor (TNF)-alpha, and C-reactive protein (CRP), are linked to stress related disorders such as major depression [8] and PTSD.

The association of PTSD with a pro-inflammatory activation of the immune system may contribute to accelerated aging [9]. PTSD has shown an association with aging, cardiovascular disease [10] autoimmune disorders and dementia [11]. In this chapter we review the reports from the translational studies about chemokines in PTSD of military service members. The translational research provides not only a better understanding of the molecular mechanisms of the devastating stress–related disorders, but also the knowledge for developing a possible diagnostic approach beneficial to both civilians and military service members.

2. Cytokine and stress-related disorders, PTSD and depression

Substantial evidence demonstrates that PTSD is associated with cytokine dysfunction. For example, patients with PTSD have higher serum cytokine concentrations than those without PTSD in anti-CCP positive rheumatoid arthritis (RA) subjects [12]. PTSD has significantly higher levels of interleukin (IL)-1β, IL-6 and tumor necrosis factor (TNF)-α peripheral blood mononuclear cells (PBMCs). The elevated levels are also associated with PTSD symptom severity [13].

Increased levels of cytokines may activate some neurotransmitter pathways reducing growth factor concentrations while producing changes in monoamines, glutamate, and other peptide transmitters. The cytokines themselves may be the result of environmental factors or psychiatric stress such as trauma during childhood, current stress, sleep disorder. Chronic stress results in upregulated cytokines, which dysregulate the neurotransmitter and cellular signal transduction leading to depression and other diseases [14]. Cytokines are able to go through the brain-barrier [15] Peripheral cytokine levels may reflect central action and be associated with symptoms of depression and anxiety [16]. Depressed patients without medical illness and who respond poorly to antidepressants have higher circulating inflammatory cytokine levels. Their traumatic childhood experiences may play a role in their later chronic inflammation and depressive condition. The association of pro-inflammatory cytokines with degenerative processes indicates that depressive disorders may have or enhance analogous functions in the systemic immune system [17, 18].

3. PTSD and chemokines in service members

A recent study found that chemokines, a family of small cytokines [19] were associated with stress-related disorders including PTSD [12, 20]. Chemokines are chemotactic factors regulating the migration of peripheral immune cells – an action, likely relevant to the pro-inflammatory cascades [19]. In addition to chemotaxis, chemokines potentiate and activate peripheral immune cells to direct the pro-inflammatory activation state, contributing to the neurodegenerative and pro-apoptotic cascades often seen in depression and Alzheimer's disease [21–24]. For example, CXCL11 is associated with aging-related impairment, including impairment of hippocampal neurogenesis, learning and memory [25]. Early evidence suggests novel non-immune and CNS-specific mechanisms of chemokines, including neuromodulation, neuroendocrine regulation, and direct neurotransmitter-like actions [26–28]. Moreover, an animal study shows that chemokine receptor (CCR6, CCR7, CXCR5) knockout mice demonstrate psychiatric- and neurobiological- like behaviors [29–31].

Chemokines regulate leukocyte migration and positioning though their receptors, which are expressed on the target cell surface [32]. Their molecular weight is 8–13 kDa. Their receptors are typical G protein-coupled transmembrane proteins, which may bind multiple ligands with variable affinity [19, 33]. There are about 44 chemokines, which are categorized into four different families (CC, CXC, CX3C, C) according to their biological behavior and structure. They regulate intracellular signaling leading to increased intracellular calcium [34] and may directly interact with G-protein-coupled receptors [35]. They also regulate the release of pro-inflammatory mediators and control of T-helper (Th)-1/Th-2 phenotypic polarization [33, 36]. Their receptor expression is observed in the brain [37–40]. Certain chemokines, such as CCL2, CCL3, CCL19, CCL21, CXCL8, CXCL12, and CX3CL1, are expressed under physiological conditions [40], while other may be expressed and upregulated in response to injury or inflammation.

The diversity of accordance and severity of PTSD symptoms following exposure to traumatic events has been a challenge for PTSD research. The mechanism underlying the diversity of PTSD symptoms with the passage of time involves a complicated course including stress response and resilience. This perspective has important implications for chemokine marker research, which is related to not only the underlying PTSD pathology, but also the dysregulation and abnormalities of immune function following exposure to traumatic stress. Recently, a prospective cohort study (paired and non-paired, pre- and post-deployment design) found [41] seven dysregulated chemokines biomarkers for PTSD, including 5CC (CCL2, CCL15, CCL23, CCL22 and CCL25,) and 2 CXC (CXCL2 and CXCL12), five possible PTSD risk markers, four stress response markers and one resilience marker (**Figure 1**).

As disease biomarkers for PTSD, 5CC (CCL2, CCL15, CCL23, CCL22 and CCL25,), and 2 CXC (CXCL2 and CXCL12) have been found dysregulated. Among them, CCL2, CCL22, CCL15, and CXCL2 were significantly upregulated, while CCL25 and CXCL12 were downregulated, in subjects with PTSD.

Considering stress response, potential chemokine markers response include CCL3 and CXCL5 which have been shown to be downregulation, while the markers CXCL 11 and CXCL16 have been shown to be up-regulated. Moreover, as risk markers for PTSD, CCL13, CCL23 and CXCL6 levels were lower pre-deployment in solders who developed PTSD than in control pre-deployment. But, CCL20 was significantly higher in the case of pre- deployment than in the control pre-deployment soldiers. Differences of CCL23 levels were also identified between PTSD pre-deployment and PTSD post-deployment, indicating there is an overlap of CCL23 dysregulation among the control, non-PTSD, case control and case. Therefore, it may be a "sticky" marker for subjects at PTSD risk or with PTSD.

CX3CL1 has been identified as a possible resilience marker (comparing the levels of chemokines between PTSD at post-deployment and non-PTSD of

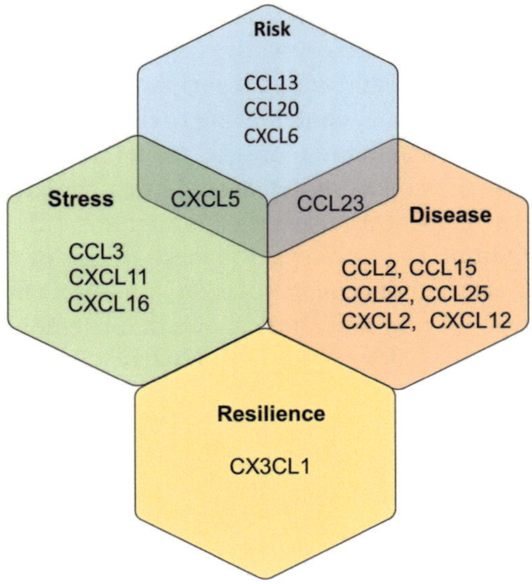

Figure 1.
Venn diagram showing potential chemokine markers for PTSD occurrence, risk, and resilience, as well as stress response. The overlap of two potential chemokine markers (CXCL5 and CCL23) is also shown.

post-deployment). CX3CL1 was not significantly different between controls at pre-deployment and controls at post-deployment. The data indicate that although deployment resulted in an up-regulation of CX3CL1 in soldiers with PTSD prior to deployment (case pre- vs. case post-), it did not alter the basal levels of CX3CL1 in non-PTSD controls (control pre- vs. control post-). Therefore CX3CL1 may be a potential resilience marker [20].

The four subgroups of chemokines are listed in **Table 1**: CXC, CC, CX3C and C. There are two adjacent cysteines (amino acids), near their amino terminus in the CC chemokine (or β-chemokine) proteins. The two N-terminal cysteines of CXC chemokines (or α-chemokines) are separated by one amino acid, represented in this name with an "X". Unlike all other chemokines C chemokines have only two cysteines; one N-terminal cysteine and one cysteine downstream. A fourth group CX3C has three amino acids between the two cysteines. CX3CL1 is only CX3C chemokine discovered. It is a chemoattractant and serves as an adhesion molecule. **Table 1** shows the summary of subgroup of chemokines which are potential markers for PTSD: onset, risk and resilience as well as stress response. **Figure 2** demonstrates subgroups of chemokine as different markers. These results warrant further systematic analytical and clinical validation research.

Dysregulation of the immune system in the stress response has long been considered a remarkable abnormal physiologic process in PTSD and stress associated disorders in service members and veterans [42, 43]. For example veterans coming back from the Gulf War have been reported to be more likely to suffer from rheumatism [44], sarcoidosis and multiple sclerosis suggesting that immunological changes may be involved in the occurrence and maintenance of PTSD (https://www.livescience.com/8916-battle-7-health-problems-facing-veterans.html). Cytokine/chemokine biomarkers have also been specifically associated with Gulf War Illness (GWI) in military population [45–47]. In a provocative study of PBMCs of chronic fatigue syndrome (CFS) subjects, over 60% of the CFS patients had DNA from a human gammaretrovirus, xenotropic murine leukemia virus-related virus (XMRV) while only 3.7% were identified in controls. Moreover, patient-derived XMRV was infectious [47], indicating it is possible that XMRV may be a contributing factor in the immune responses or pathogenesis of CFS. In addition, it has also

Markers	PTSD	Stress response	PTSD risk	Resilience
Chemokines				
CC	CCL2	CCL3	CCL13	
	CCL15		CCL20	
	CCL22		CCL23	
	CCL23			
	CCL25			
CXC	CXCL2	CXCL5	CXCL5	
	CXCL12	CXCL11	CXCL6	
		CXCL16		
CX3C				CX3CL1
C				

Table 1.
Summary of subgroups of potential chemokine markers for PTSD, PTSD risk and resilience, as well as stress response.

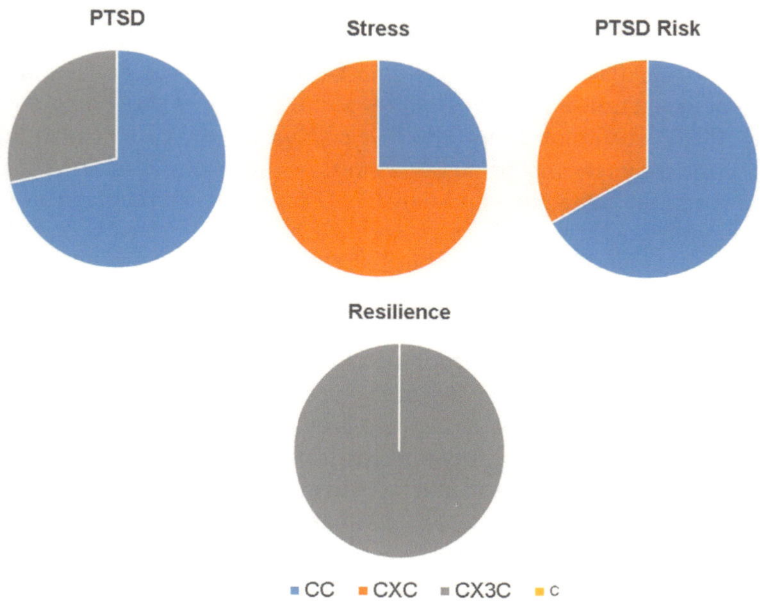

Figure 2.
Distribution of subgroups of chemokines as different markers as found in our previous study. Findings suggest that 15 out of 40 chemokines are differentially associated with PTSD, PTSD risk, stress-responses and resilience.

been reported that GWI patients had higher lymphocyte, monocyte, neutrophil, and platelet counts compared with controls. The six serum proteins of inflammation were also significantly different from controls including C reactive protein [45]. The results suggest that inflammation is a component of the pathobiology of GWI in the veterans.

Some studies have suggested that the risk of autoimmune disorders in PTSD is higher in psychiatric subjects than in those with no psychiatric diagnosis [48]. Interferons (INF)s, interleukins (ILs), lymphokines, tumor necrosis factor (TNF), which are often altered in response to an immune stimulus are involved in regulation of immunity and inflammation [9–11]. PTSD may have higher levels of certain cytokines (IL-2, IL-4, IL-6, IL-8, IL-10 and TNF-α) than age- and gender-matched healthy controls, suggesting a generalized inflammatory state in PTSD [49]. Experimental endotoxin injection up-regulates plasma IL6, IL-10, and TNF-α, which has been associated with depression-like symptoms often seen in PTSD [50]. However, the results of cytokine levels in PTSD are mixed. While some reports show that PTSD patients had higher levels of IL-1β [51], IL-6, and TNF-α in the plasma [52], other reports no significant difference in levels of IL-1β [53] and IL-6 [53, 54] and IL-8 [54] between PTSD and controls [55]. These inconsistent findings may be partially attributable to variation of study subjects including differences of traumatic events (e.g. childhood vs. adulthood), the trauma duration (e.g. Life time vs. current), samples from different population (general population vs. service members), differences of geography and treatment (with or without), and testing approaches (ELISA vs. Western blot, and blood vs. saliva or CSF).

In our recent chemokine study, we used a prospective study design and collected PCL scores and blood samples from US soldiers pre- and post-deployment (pre-, post-) to a war zone during the Iraq and Afghanistan. We examined multiple (40) chemokines using luminex assay (a high-throughput biochip). All subjects experienced deployment to the war. The controls were not only self- but also age- and sex-matched. All subjects were at the same location (Guam) and was also Reserve or National Guard who had no medication. Our hypothesis we tested was that deployment stressful life events area associated with PTSD and chemokine/cytokine biomarkers. Potential disease markers, the blood chemokines, showed significant differences between PTSD cases pre- and post-; different basal levels of blood chemokine between non-PTSD control pre- and PTSD cases pre- being the risk markers for PTSD; different chemokine levels between non-PTSD controls pre- and non-PTSD controls post- may be possible stress response markers, and the differences between PTSD cases post- and non-PTSD controls post representing possible markers for resilience.

In recent years, cytokine detection and quantification has served as an important tool in biomarker research due to the capacity of simultaneous measurements of multiple cytokines in a single run in a small sample size. Simultaneous measurements of multiple blood cytokines provide an experimental strategy resolving complex interactions among signaling molecules to obtain a pattern of numerous cytokines within an experiment. It may also provide a more inclusive and comprehensive depiction of the association of cytokines with PTSD. It appears to be better than conventional assays such as ELISA, which measures individual cytokine only [20]. In addition, a prospective research design is important [41]. These factors make the study of chemokines/cytokines more significant for determining (their association with PTSD).

4. Concluding remarks

Although studies show cytokines and chemokines are associated with stress-related conditions, such as depression and PTSD particularly in the military population, the results sometimes are inconclusive. The study of chemokine biomarkers for PTSD is still in its early stages. Current studies suggest there is an excess of inflammatory action of the immune system in PTSD, which is linked to PTSD vulnerability. It is possible that dysregulation of cortisol plays an important role in this excessive inflammation. Moreover, accumulating evidence both at the bench and in the clinic indicate that dysregulated chemokines are potential molecular targets for diagnosis and treatment of PTSD. Potential chemokine biomarkers associated with PTSD onset, risk and resilience as well as other stress responses have been identified in military population (**Figure 1**). Translational research in service members leads some support to the idea that altered chemokine expression may contribute to PTSD pathophysiology. This may in turn provide an opportunity to identify chemokine biomarkers not only for PTSD onset, risk, and resilience, but also other stress-responses as well.

Funding, declaration of interest, and acknowledgements

This study was funded by Center for the Study of Traumatic Stress. All authors declare no conflict of interest. The authors thank to Hieu Dinh, and Luna Zhang for their editing of the paper.

Disclaimer statement

The opinions and assertions expressed herein are those of the author(s) and do not necessarily reflect the official policy or position of the Uniformed Services University or the Department of Defense.

Author details

Lei Zhang*, Xianzhang Hu, Xiaoxia Li and Robert J. Ursano
Center for the Study of Traumatic Stress, Department of Psychiatry, Uniformed Services University of the Health Sciences, Bethesda, MD, USA

*Address all correspondence to: lezhang@usuhs.edu

References

[1] Richardson, L.K., B.C. Frueh, and R. Acierno, *Prevalence estimates of combat-related post-traumatic stress disorder: critical review.* Aust N Z J Psychiatry, 2010. **44**(1): p. 4-19.

[2] Jonas, D.E., et al., in *Psychological and Pharmacological Treatments for Adults With Posttraumatic Stress Disorder (PTSD)*. 2013: Rockville (MD).

[3] Bisson, J.I., et al., *Psychological therapies for chronic post-traumatic stress disorder (PTSD) in adults.* Cochrane Database Syst Rev, 2013(12): p. CD003388.

[4] Davis, A.K., et al., *Psychedelic Treatment for Trauma-Related Psychological and Cognitive Impairment Among US Special Operations Forces Veterans.* Chronic Stress, 2020. **4**: p. 2470547020939564.

[5] Hetrick, S.E., et al., *Combined pharmacotherapy and psychological therapies for post traumatic stress disorder (PTSD).* Cochrane Database Syst Rev, 2010(7): p. CD007316.

[6] Stein, M.B., et al., *Genome-wide association analyses of post-traumatic stress disorder and its symptom subdomains in the Million Veteran Program.* Nature Genetics, 2021.

[7] Licinio, J. and M.L. Wong, *Launching the 'War on Mental Illness'.* Molecular Psychiatry, 2014. **19**(1): p. 1-5.

[8] Lanquillon, S., et al., *Cytokine production and treatment response in major depressive disorder.* Neuropsychopharmacology, 2000. **22**(4): p. 370-379.

[9] Hori, H. and Y. Kim, *Inflammation and post-traumatic stress disorder.* Psychiatry Clin Neurosci, 2019. **73**(4): p. 143-153.

[10] Song, H., et al., *Stress related disorders and risk of cardiovascular disease: population based, sibling controlled cohort study.* BMJ (Clinical research ed.), 2019. **365**: p. l1850-l1850.

[11] Liu, J., J. Lu, and X. Luo, *Stress-Related Disorders and Autoimmune Disease.* JAMA, 2018. **320**(17): p. 1816-1817.

[12] Maloley, P.M., et al., *Post-traumatic stress disorder and serum cytokine and chemokine concentrations in patients with rheumatoid arthritis(☆).* Semin Arthritis Rheum, 2019. **49**(2): p. 229-235.

[13] Gola, H., et al., *Posttraumatic stress disorder is associated with an enhanced spontaneous production of pro-inflammatory cytokines by peripheral blood mononuclear cells.* BMC Psychiatry, 2013. **13**: p. 40.

[14] Kronfol, Z. and D.G. Remick, *Cytokines and the brain: implications for clinical psychiatry.* Am J Psychiatry, 2000. **157**(5): p. 683-694.

[15] Banks, W.A., A.J. Kastin, and R.D. Broadwell, *Passage of cytokines across the blood-brain barrier.* Neuroimmunomodulation, 1995. **2**(4): p. 241-248.

[16] Martinez, P., et al., *Circulating cytokine levels are associated with symptoms of depression and anxiety among people with alcohol and drug use disorders.* J Neuroimmunol, 2018. **318**: p. 80-86.

[17] Dantzer, R., et al., *From inflammation to sickness and depression: when the immune system subjugates the brain.* Nature reviews. Neuroscience, 2008. **9**(1): p. 46-56.

[18] Eyre, H. and B.T. Baune, *Neuroplastic changes in depression:*

a role for the immune system. Psychoneuroendocrinology, 2012. **37**(9): p. 1397-1416.

[19] Murphy, P.M., et al., *International union of pharmacology. XXII. Nomenclature for chemokine receptors.* Pharmacol Rev, 2000. **52**(1): p. 145-176.

[20] Zhang, L., et al., *The interaction between stressful life events and leukocyte telomere length is associated with PTSD.* Mol Psychiatry, 2014. **19**(8): p. 855-856.

[21] Ono, S.J., et al., *Chemokines: roles in leukocyte development, trafficking, and effector function.* J Allergy Clin Immunol, 2003. **111**(6): p. 1185-1199; quiz 1200.

[22] Le, Y., et al., *Chemokines and chemokine receptors: their manifold roles in homeostasis and disease.* Cell Mol Immunol, 2004. **1**(2): p. 95-104.

[23] Moylan, S., et al., *The neuroprogressive nature of major depressive disorder: pathways to disease evolution and resistance, and therapeutic implications.* Mol Psychiatry, 2013. **18**(5): p. 595-606.

[24] Jo, W.K., A.C. Law, and S.K. Chung, *The neglected co-star in the dementia drama: the putative roles of astrocytes in the pathogeneses of major neurocognitive disorders.* Mol Psychiatry, 2014. **19**(2): p. 159-167.

[25] Villeda, S.A., et al., *The ageing systemic milieu negatively regulates neurogenesis and cognitive function.* Nature, 2011. **477**(7362): p. 90-94.

[26] Rostène, W., P. Kitabgi, and S.M. Parsadaniantz, *Chemokines: a new class of neuromodulator?* Nat Rev Neurosci, 2007. **8**(11): p. 895-903.

[27] Rostène, W., et al., *Chemokines and chemokine receptors: new actors in neuroendocrine regulations.* Front Neuroendocrinol, 2011. **32**(1): p. 10-24.

[28] Réaux-Le Goazigo, A., et al., *Current status of chemokines in the adult CNS.* Prog Neurobiol, 2013. **104**: p. 67-92.

[29] Harrison, E.L., et al., *Maternal separation modifies behavioural and neuroendocrine responses to stress in CCR7 deficient mice.* Behav Brain Res, 2014. **263**: p. 169-175.

[30] Jaehne, E.J. and B.T. Baune, *Effects of chemokine receptor signalling on cognition-like, emotion-like and sociability behaviours of CCR6 and CCR7 knockout mice.* Behav Brain Res, 2014. **261**: p. 31-39.

[31] Stuart, M.J., F. Corrigan, and B.T. Baune, *Knockout of CXCR5 increases the population of immature neural cells and decreases proliferation in the hippocampal dentate gyrus.* J Neuroinflammation, 2014. **11**: p. 31.

[32] Morteau, O., *CHEMOKINES*, in *Encyclopedia of Respiratory Medicine*, G.J. Laurent and S.D. Shapiro, Editors. 2006, Academic Press: Oxford. p. 356-365.

[33] Cyster, J.G., *Chemokines and cell migration in secondary lymphoid organs.* Science, 1999. **286**(5447): p. 2098-2102.

[34] Nelson, T.E. and D.L. Gruol, *The chemokine CXCL10 modulates excitatory activity and intracellular calcium signaling in cultured hippocampal neurons.* J Neuroimmunol, 2004. **156**(1-2): p. 74-87.

[35] Baggiolini, M., B. Dewald, and B. Moser, *Human chemokines: an update.* Annu Rev Immunol, 1997. **15**: p. 675-705.

[36] Rossi, D. and A. Zlotnik, *The biology of chemokines and their receptors.* Annu Rev Immunol, 2000. **18**: p. 217-242.

[37] Bajetto, A., et al., *Chemokines and their receptors in the central nervous system.* Front Neuroendocrinol, 2001. **22**(3): p. 147-184.

[38] Miller, R.J., et al., *Chemokine action in the nervous system.* J Neurosci, 2008. **28**(46): p. 11792-11795.

[39] Rostène, W., et al., *Neurochemokines: a menage a trois providing new insights on the functions of chemokines in the central nervous system.* J Neurochem, 2011. **118**(5): p. 680-694.

[40] Jaerve, A. and H.W. Müller, *Chemokines in CNS injury and repair.* Cell Tissue Res, 2012. **349**(1): p. 229-248.

[41] Zhang, L., et al., *Potential chemokine biomarkers associated with PTSD onset, risk and resilience as well as stress responses in US military service members.* Translational Psychiatry, 2020. **10**(1): p. 31.

[42] Khansari, D.N., A.J. Murgo, and R.E. Faith, *Effects of stress on the immune system.* Immunology today, 1990. **11**(5): p. 170-175.

[43] Dantzer, R. and K.W. Kelley, *Stress and immunity: an integrated view of relationships between the brain and the immune system.* Life sciences, 1989. **44**(26): p. 1995-2008.

[44] Grady, E.P., et al., *Rheumatic findings in Gulf War veterans.* Arch Intern Med, 1998. **158**(4): p. 367-371.

[45] Johnson, G.J., et al., *Blood Biomarkers of Chronic Inflammation in Gulf War Illness.* PLoS One, 2016. **11**(6): p. e0157855.

[46] Broderick, G., et al., *Exploring the Diagnostic Potential of Immune Biomarker Co-expression in Gulf War Illness.* Methods Mol Biol, 2018. **1781**: p. 101-120.

[47] Lombardi, V.C., et al., *Detection of an infectious retrovirus, XMRV, in blood cells of patients with chronic fatigue syndrome.* Science, 2009. **326**(5952): p. 585-589.

[48] O'Donovan, A., et al., *Elevated risk for autoimmune disorders in iraq and afghanistan veterans with posttraumatic stress disorder.* Biol Psychiatry, 2015. **77**(4): p. 365-374.

[49] Guo, M., et al., *Study on serum cytokine levels in posttraumatic stress disorder patients.* Asian Pac J Trop Med, 2012. **5**(4): p. 323-325.

[50] Grigoleit, J.S., et al., *Dose-dependent effects of endotoxin on neurobehavioral functions in humans.* PLoS One, 2011. **6**(12): p. e28330.

[51] Wang, W., et al., *Characteristics of pro- and anti-inflammatory cytokines alteration in PTSD patients exposed to a deadly earthquake.* J Affect Disord, 2019. **248**: p. 52-58.

[52] Hori, H., et al., *Proinflammatory status-stratified blood transcriptome profiling of civilian women with PTSD.* Psychoneuroendocrinology, 2020. **111**: p. 104491.

[53] von Kanel, R., et al., *Evidence for low-grade systemic proinflammatory activity in patients with posttraumatic stress disorder.* J Psychiatr Res, 2007. **41**(9): p. 744-752.

[54] Song, Y., et al., *Disturbance of serum interleukin-2 and interleukin-8 levels in posttraumatic and non-posttraumatic stress disorder earthquake survivors in northern China.* Neuroimmunomodulation, 2007. **14**(5): p. 248-254.

[55] Lindqvist, D., et al., *Proinflammatory milieu in combat-related PTSD is independent of depression and early life stress.* Brain Behav Immun, 2014. **42**: p. 81-88.

Chapter 4

Combat Casualty Care for Children: *Peculiarities, Problems, and Provisions*

Sunil Jain

Abstract

Armed Forces doctors are often required to treat children affected in war, combat, and disasters. Tender care & comprehensive tact is needed for children. Acquisition of these qualities comes with knowledge, its application, and practicing skills. Throughout history, children have been victims of armed conflict. War-related injuries are more severe as compared to the civilian sector injuries. Penetrating injuries are associated with significant damage to local structures, whereas blast injuries are associated with less local injury and more multisystem trauma. Children are not small adults. The differences have important practice implications. Identifying and correcting physiological compromise improves outcomes. The examination and vital sign data can be interpreted only if the caregiver has a thorough understanding of normal values. Identification & treatment of what is killing the patient is done in primary survey. Secondary survey, extremity trauma, fracture biomechanics, & burns peculiarities need attention. Care of the injured patient is a dynamic process. Frequent monitoring required for proper response. Small infants have a narrow margin for error. Combat trauma provides multiple opportunities for improvement. Continuation of research will ensure ongoing progress and further improvement in the outcomes of both military and civilian casualties.

Keywords: pediatric, combat care, multiple trauma, battlefield resuscitation, transfusion protocols, burns

1. Introduction

The scenario & statistics are highly suggestive of the need for heightened professionalism in treating children affected in war, combat, and disasters. Armed Forces doctors are often required to treat these children.

Throughout history, children have been victims of armed conflict. War-related injuries tend to be more severe as compared to the civilian sector [1]. In children combat-related injuries have a higher mortality than noncombat injuries or other admissions [2].

The primary mission of the Armed Forces field hospitals deployed in support of combat operations is 'The care of its injured troops". However they often provide care to civilians including pediatric patients [3]. Children are treated for combat injuries and also non-combat conditions on humanitarian grounds.

The reported workload of children treated in Armed Forces field hospitals recently ranged from 4–25% in various studies [4–7]. A study of pediatric casualties treated in U.S. and coalition military hospitals in Iraq and Afghanistan has reported that majority require intensive care [8].

Tender care & comprehensive tact is needed for children. Acquisition of these qualities comes with knowledge, its application, and practicing skills. Experiences from recent wars and disasters have highlighted the surgeons' increasingly crucial role in these scenarios. Surgeons should attend Advanced Trauma Life Support (ATLS) programme which covers trauma in children [9]. *Matos et al* have commented that "*Providing forward-deployed medical staff with training in the acute care of young children with severe traumatic injuries may improve outcomes in this population*" [10].

The Committee on Tactical Combat Casualty Care (TCCC), Joint Trauma System, U.S. Army Institute of Surgical Research has commented "*TCCC has taken a leadership role in advocating for battlefield trauma care advances*" [11]. TCCC is essentially a set of best-practice guidelines of pre-hospital trauma care customized for use in the battlefield. It includes (i) tourniquets and hemostatic dressings: aggressive use to control life-threatening external hemorrhage; (ii) fluid resuscitation: improved protocols and techniques for casualties in hemorrhagic shock; (iii) airway positioning and surgical airways: increased emphasis on these to manage the traumatized airway; (iv) battlefield analgesia: faster, safer, and more effective; (v) intra-osseous vascular access: increased use when needed; (vi) battlefield antibiotics; (vii) good medicine with good small-unit tactics combination [11]. The good of small victims – the children, can be greatly done with good understanding and the elaboration done below of pertinent specific challenges and professional special care.

2. Anatomical and physiological peculiarities

2.1 Adults vs. children

- Children are not small adults. Their anatomy and physiology is different. The differences have important implications for surgical practice.

- Children are more prone to multiple trauma [12]. This is logical given the same damaging force and small body size. Further the smaller body size in children results in a greater force applied per unit surface area (in blast injuries) /weight (in penetrating injuries). The energy is transmitted to a body with less fat, less connective tissue, and an immature skeleton; therefore injuries to multiple organs are more frequent.

- Pediatric airway is not a miniature replica of adult airway. It has different anatomy with regards to proportion and angulation. In pediatric population, epiglottis is large, floppy and omega-shaped. It makes an angle of 45° with the base of tongue. At birth, larynx is situated opposite to the lower border of C4 vertebra. It descends to C4–C5 interspace by the age of 3 years and finally descends to lie opposite to the body of C5. Importantly, the tonsils and adenoids appear in the second year of life and generally reach their largest size by 4–7 years, posing a risk of obstruction [13].

- Children are more susceptible to hypothermia. In children the surface area to body volume ratio is high. They have less subcutaneous fat, immature vasomotor control, and greater heat loss from pulmonary evaporation. This results in a higher thermal energy loss, necessitating guarding against hypothermia.

2.2 Injury patterns

- Children are commonly injured and sustain more severe injuries [14]. Young pediatric patients (ages ≤8 years) compared with older pediatric and adult patients have been reported to have increased severity of injury, as indicated by decreased Glasgow Coma Scale score; increased incidence of hypotension, base deficit, and serum pH on admission; red blood cell transfusion requirements; and increased injury severity scores on admission [10].

- Penetrating injuries are associated with significant damage to local structures, whereas blast injuries are associated with less local injury and more multisystem trauma [15].

- Young children have relatively large heads with immature neck musculature. This results in more susceptibility to cervical spine injury caused by the fulcrum effect in the C1–C3 area. Children under age 8 years are also susceptible to SCIWORA (spinal cord injury without radiographic abnormality).

- A child's chest wall is relatively pliable, therefore less force is absorbed by the rib cage & more is transmitted to the lungs. This makes pulmonary contusions frequent in children with blunt chest trauma. Children have more mobile mediastinal structures. Thus, a tension pneumothorax can shift the mediastinum causing respiratory & cardio-vascular compromise. It should always be considered in hypotensive-hypoxic child. It should also be noted that in children the thorax is disproportionately smaller as compared to the cranium and abdomen, hence if thoracic trauma is present one must assess the entire patient to rule out Traumatic Brain Injuries and abdominal injuries

- Infants & small children have a wider abdomen, a broader costal margin & a shallower pelvis. This makes liver, spleen & bladder trauma more common. In children the smaller & more pliable ribs offer less protection than those in adults. The spleen & liver are the organs most vulnerable to injury from blunt- or penetrating-force trauma.

2.3 Physiological parameters

- Identifying and correcting physiological compromise improves outcomes.

- Physiologically Total Body Water (TBW) as a percentage of body weight varies with age. TBW is 75% of body weight in a term infant. In the first year of life TBW decreases to approximately 60% of body weight and remains at this level until puberty. At puberty TBW changes are different in females and males. The fat content of females increases more than that of males. Males acquire more muscle mass than females. Fat has very low water content and muscle has high water content. Hence by the end of puberty, TBW remains at 60% in males, but in females it decreases to approximately 50% of body weight. Also the high fat content in overweight children causes a decrease in TBW as a percentage of body weight.

- Body weight is a critical measurement in children, because this is a major determinant of fluid balance and drug doses. At the turn of the century a peacetime study reported that incorrect recording of patient weights leading to an incorrect medication dose is a common cause for medication errors in the pediatric emergency department [16]. Estimation methods are useful in emergencies. A Tactical Combat Casualty Care oriented Broselow tape relates a child's height as measured by the tape to his/her weight to provide medical instructions. These include medication dosages, the size of the equipment that should be used, and the level of shock voltage when using a defibrillator.

- Vital signs are vital in detecting and assessing physiologic instability. These vary with age, & normal are:

Age	Heart rate (beats/minute)	Blood pressure (mm Hg)	Respiratory rate (breaths/min)
Premature	120–170	55–75/35–45	40–70
0–3 mths	100–150	65–85/45–55	35–55
3–6 mths	90–120	70–90/50–65	30–45
6–12 mths	80–120	80–100/55–65	25–40
1–3 yrs	70–110	90–105/55–70	20–30
3–6 yrs	65–110	95–110/60–75	20–25
6-12 yrs	60–95	100–120/60–75	14–22
12 yrs	55–85	110–135/65–85	12–18

Practical principles of use:

- child's respiratory rate should not be >60breaths/min for a sustained period;
- normal heart rate is 2–3 times normal respiratory rate for age; and
- pediatric blood pressure simple assessment: the lower limit of systolic blood pressure should be:

≥60 mm Hg for neonates;
≥70 mm Hg for 1 mo-1 yr. olds;
≥70 mm Hg + (2 × age) for 1–10 yr. olds; and
≥90 mm Hg for any child older than 10 yr.

Values not meeting these criteria are pathological.

- The examination and vital sign data can be interpreted only if the caregiver has a thorough understanding of normal values.
- All deviations from these physiological norms are pathological and need to be suitably corrected.

3. Battlefield resuscitation

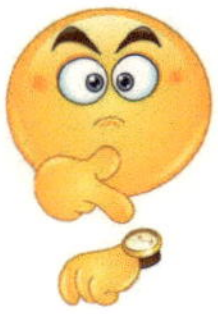

The principles of ATLS should be followed. The philosophy of this is to identify & treat what is killing the patient in the primary survey. In the secondary survey one should proceed to identify all other injuries.

The trend evolving lays stress on correcting the physiological derangement, with surgical intervention restricted to stopping any active surgical bleeding & controlling any contamination.

3.1 Primary survey

- This addresses the ABCDEs: **a**irway, **b**reathing, **c**irculation, neurologic **d**eficit, & **e**xposure of patient & control of **e**nvironment.

3.1.1 Airway

- Optimizing oxygenation and ventilation while protecting the cervical spine from potential further injury is of paramount importance. Any child with multiple trauma should be suspected of having a cervical spine injury. Children are at risk for such injuries because of their large heads, which augment flexion-extension forces, and weak neck muscles, which predispose them to ligament injuries. If it is necessary to open the airway, a jaw thrust without head tilt is recommended. This procedure minimizes cervical spine motion. During maintenance of the airway it is important not to overextend the neck as this can lead to respiratory obstruction because of shorter neck and relatively larger tongue in children.

3.1.2 Breathing

- This should be assessed with the respiratory rate; visualizing chest wall motion for symmetry, depth and accessory muscle use; and auscultating breath sounds in both axillae. If breathing is inadequate, bag-valve-mask ventilation with 100% oxygen must be initiated immediately followed by endotracheal intubation. While intubating a child the following anatomical peculiarities of the airway in children should be borne in mind: smaller; more anteriorly placed, more difficult to visualize; and more prone to prone to mucosal injuries, leading to subglottic stenosis. The formulas for selecting the appropriate size ETT & its insertion are:

  Uncuffed ETT size (mm) = (age in yrs/4) + 4
  Cuffed ETT size (mm) = (age in yrs/4) + 3.5
  ETT depth (from lip to mid-trahea) = ETT internal diameter (size) x 3

- In the field, competent bag-mask ventilation may be preferable. Endotracheal intubation should be performed only by skilled providers.

A view from the history

- A substantial amount of medical and surgical progress has emanated from experiences in the battlefield. Sir Ivan Whiteside Magill developed the endotracheal tube during the First World War to facilitate plastic surgery around the mouth. It is pertinent to quote here:

  "*Necessity is the mother of invention, but for the Armed Forces*
  Adversity is the mother of all improvisations, innovations and inventions".

- Further dealing with pediatric patients in the battlefield, which is even more challenging task, should lead to more improvisations, innovations and inventions.

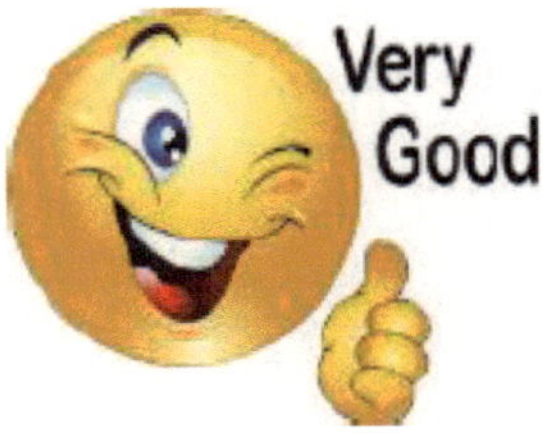

3.1.3 Circulation

- In children rapid thready pulse is a more reliable and earlier warning sign than a fall in blood pressure. More subtle signs need to be looked for early diagnosis. These are weakened or loss of peripheral pulse, reduced capillary refill, mottled pale skin, cooled extremities, reduced pulse pressure and changes in mentation.

- Blood pressure remains normal in early shock, as body compensates by increase in heart rate and peripheral vascular resistance. Blood pressure declines with loss of more than 25% of the blood volume. For a child weighing 10 kg this is only 200 ml! (20 ml/kg). With losses >25% hypotension ensues. Hypotension is a late and ominous sign of hypovolemic shock.

- Intravenous (IV) access is important and the quickest way to achieve is cannulating a larger vein, such as an ante-cubital vein. In a severely injured child, a 2nd catheter should be placed within the first few minutes of resuscitation. If IV access proves difficult readily and rapidly, an intra-osseous catheter is next option. All medications and fluids can be administered intra-osseously. *Cooper et al* have used this effectively in combat casualty care. They used IO needles to administer fluid (crystalloid, packed red cells and fresh frozen plasma) and drugs (analgesics, cardiac arrest drugs, antibiotics, drugs for both rapid sequence induction and maintenance of anesthesia) [17]. Next alternatives include central venous access using the Seldinger technique (femoral vein) or surgical cutdown (saphenous vein).

- A portable ultrasonic device may be of great help in locating and cannulating veins, especially those of the neck and groin.

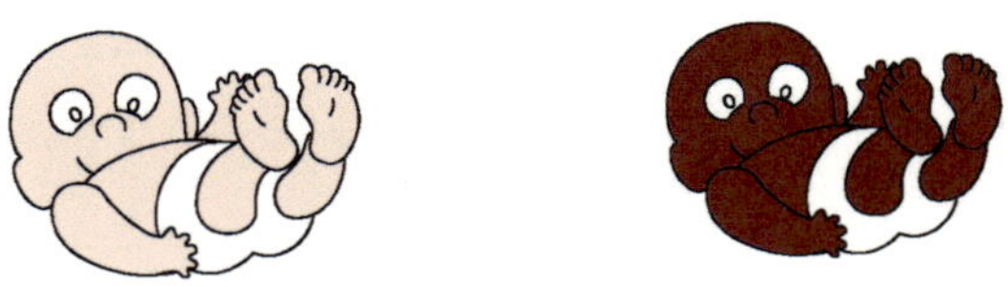

- Patients with on-going hemodynamic instability require prompt intervention. In shock, early aggressive intravenous fluid resuscitation is essential to prevent further deterioration. Isotonic crystalloid solution- Ringer lactate or normal saline (20 ml/kg) should be infused rapidly. If necessary, crystalloid boluses should be repeated. Most children stabilize with administration of crystalloid solution alone. However if patient remains in shock after boluses totaling

40–60 ml/kg of crystalloid then 10-15 ml/kg of cross-matched packed red blood cells should be transfused. Early initiation of massive transfusion protocols (including fresh-frozen plasma) prevents coagulopathy. If shock persists despite these measures, surgery to stop internal hemorrhage is usually indicated.

- Frequent monitoring required for proper response. Small infants have a narrow margin for error.

- Severe combat injuries frequently require massive transfusion of large volumes of blood products. Experience from numerous military accounts in Iraq and Afghanistan indicates that patients receiving equal or near equal ratios of packed red blood cells to fresh frozen plasma and platelets had increased survival [18–21].

3.1.4 Neurologic deficit

- In the primary survey, neurologic status is briefly assessed using by evaluating the level of conciousness and determining pupil size and reactivity. Different assessment and monitoring tool can be used. The level of consciousness can be classified using the mnemonic ***AVPU***: **A**lert, responsive to **V**erbal commands, responsive to **P**ainful stimuli, or **U**nresponsive, details at **Table 1** [22]. The Glasgow Coma Scale (GCS) is the most widely used method of evaluating neurologic function, details of it and useful adaptation for children is at **Table 2** [23]. Unlike the GCS, the AVPU scale is not developmentally dependent. The posture should also be looked at.

In head injuries the primary direct cerebral injury occurs within seconds of the event and is irreversible. Secondary injury is caused by subsequent anoxia or ischemia. Our goal is to minimize secondary injury by ensuring adequate oxygenation, ventilation, and perfusion, and maintaining normal intracranial pressure (ICP). A child with Glasgow Coma Score of 8 or less, benefits from ICP monitoring and should be intubated. Evaluation should be done for craniotomy.

3.1.5 Exposure and environmental control

- Exposure is the final component of the primary assessment. This is performed only after the child's airway, breathing, and circulation are stable or have been stabilized through simple interventions.

- Exposure *has to be efficient.* Purpose is to assess for previously unidentified injures. Care has to be taken that exposure in a cold environment does not cause hypothermia and cardio-pulmonary instability.

A	The child is awake, alert, and interactive with parents and care providers.
V	The child responds only if the care provider or parents call the child's name or speak loudly.
P	The child responds only to painful stimuli, such as pinching the nail bed of a toe or finger.
U	The child is unresponsive to all stimuli.

Table 1.
AVPU neurologic assessment.

EYE OPENING (TOTAL POSSIBLE POINTS 4)			
Spontaneous	4		
To voice	3		
To pain	2		
None	1		
VERBAL RESPONSE (TOTAL POSSIBLE POINTS 5)			
Older Children		**Infants and Young Children < 2 years**	
Oriented	5	Cooing/ Babbling/Appropriate words	5
Confused	4	Irritable cry	4
Inappropriate	3	Crying to pain	3
Incomprehensible	2	Moaning to pain	2
None	1	None	1
MOTOR RESPONSE (TOTAL POSSIBLE POINTS 6)			
Obeys	6		
Localizes pain	5		
Withdraws	4		
Flexion	3		
Extension	2		
None	1		

Table 2.
The Glasgow coma scale and adaptation for children.

- Temperature should be checked on arrival and monitored. If required warming is done using overhead lamps or radiant heaters as well as heated blankets and warmed intravenous fluids and blood.

3.2 The current concepts and future 🤔

- Care of the injured patient is a dynamic process. Combat trauma provides multiple opportunities for improvement [24]. Hemorrhage remains the primary cause of preventable death after trauma.

- Although literature is emerging regarding the benefits of permissive hypotension, hemostatic resuscitation, and damage control surgery for adult trauma patients, currently there is no pediatric data [25], and research needed for review and refinements of our practices.

- Balanced massive transfusion (1, 1, 1 of fresh frozen plasma, packed red blood cells, and platelets ratio) has not yet been demonstrated to have the same mortality benefits in pediatric trauma patients as in adults. Similarly, tranexamic acid (TXA) has strong evidence to support its use in adult trauma and some evidence in pediatric trauma [26].

- Further research is required for use of balanced resuscitation, massive transfusion, adjuncts such as tranexamic acid or factor VII in resuscitation in the pediatric trauma population. Technological advancements such as hemoglobin-based oxygen carriers to increase survival should also be studied.

4. Provisioning

- An ideal first aid box that will suit all terrains, all ages, & all emergencies is yet to be devised. However we should continue to improve our planning with our experiences.

- Availability of necessary equipment is a vital part of an emergency response. If in military medical appreciation treating children is anticipated then medical equipments mentioned in **Table 3** should be included. An appreciation of a situation, whether written, verbal or mental, is a logical process of reasoning & analysis leading to the best course of action. **Table 4** gives details of Pediatric Resuscitation Medications & doses. Recognition of the potential for pediatric casualties is required to facilitate appropriate planning, training & equipping of medical units deployed on future operations [27].

- Systematic planning for scientific practice should be done

- The resuscitation cart or kit should be checked regularly, for presence and functionality of its components. Out-dated medications, a laryngoscope with a failed light source or an empty oxygen tank represents a catastrophe in a resuscitation setting.

- Matos *et al* have commented that "*Providing forward-deployed medical staff with paediatric-specific equipment for the acute care of young children with severe traumatic injuries may improve outcomes in this population*" [10]. This comes from their observations of increased mortality rates of young children with traumatic injuries at a US army combat support hospital.

- Another area of concern is peri-operative and subsequent care provisioning. Both emergency and elective surgeries are performed. *Neff et al* have commented "*Elective paediatric surgical care in a forward deployed setting is feasible; however, limitations in resources for perioperative care and rehabilitation mandate prudent patient selection particularly with respect to procedures that require prolonged post-operative care*" [28].

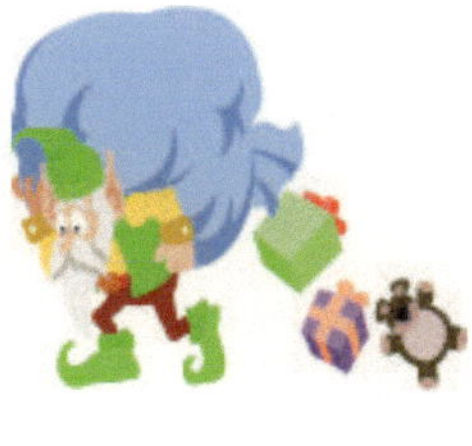

Storage cart for equipment/materials	
Airway equipment	Low pressure suction device, Yankauer tonsil tip suction, bulb syringe, suction catheters sizes 5-16F
	Oropharyngeal airways (sizes 00–5)
	Nasopharyngeal airways (sizes 12-30F)
	Magill forceps (pediatric, adult)
	Nasogastric tubes (sizes 6-14F)
	Laryngoscope handle with extra batteries, bulbs
	Laryngoscope blades– Miller straight 0, 1, 2, 3 & MacIntosh curved 2,3
	Endotracheal tubes (uncuffed 2.5–5.5; cuffed 6.0–8.0) and stylets
	Esophageal intubation detector or end-tidal carbon dioxide detector
	Nebulizer (or metered-dose inhaler with spacer/mask)
Breathing equipment	Clear oxygen masks, breather and non-rebreather, with reservoirs (infant, child, adult)
	Bag-valve-mask (450 mL and 1,000 mL)
	Oxygen and delivery system
Cardiac equipment	Cardiac arrest board for compressions
	Butterfly needles (19–25 gauge)
	Catheter-over-needle device (14–24 gauge)
	Arm boards, tape, tourniquet,
	IV adapters, T connecters, stopcocks
	Intraosseous needles (16 and 18 gauge)
	Intravenous tubing, micro-drip
	IVs, butterflies, intraosseous needles
	Tapes, alcohol, sponges
	Cutdown tray
	Umbilical catheter tray
	Defibrillator/portable ECG monitor
	Military antishock trousers kit
	Various crystalloid and colloid fluids
Monitoring equipment	Pulse oximetry, ECG, end-tidal CO_2, Sphygmomanometer (infant, child, adult, thigh cuffs)
Miscellaneous	Stiff neck collars (small/large)
	Heating source (overhead warmer/infrared lamp)
	Tactical Combat Casualty Care oriented Broselow tape
	General minor surgical procedure tray
	Tracheostomy tray
	Chest tube tray
	Pleurovac pump
	Warm packs, sandbags and so on
IV fluids	Normal saline (0.9 NS) *or* lactated Ringer solution (500 mL bags)
	5% dextrose, 0.45 NS (500 mL bags)
Medications	Albuterol for inhalation, epinephrine, antibiotics, anticonvulsants (diazepam/lorazepam), corticosteroids (parenteral/oral), dextrose (25%), diphenhydramine (parenteral), atropine, naloxone, sodium bicarbonate

Table 3.
Supplies: Pediatric emergency care.

Medication	Dose	Remarks
Atropine	• 0.02 mg/kg IV/IO • 0.03 mg/kg ET* • Repeat once if needed • Minimum dose: 0.1 mg • Minimum single dose: Child, 0.5 mg Adolescent, 1 mg	
Calcium chloride (10%)	20 mg/kg IV/IO (0.2 mL/kg)	Slowly
Calcium Gluconate (10%)	60 mg/kg IV/IO (1–2 mL/kg)	Slowly
Epinephrine	• 0.01 mg/kg (0.1 mL/kg 1: 10,000) IV/IO • 0.1 mg/kg (0.1 mL/kg 1: 1,000) ET* • Maximum dose: 1 mg IV/IO; 10 mg ET	May repeat q 3–5 min
Glucose	0.5–1 g/kg IV/IO	D10W: 5–10 mL/kg D25W: 2–4 mL/kg D50W: 1–2 mL/kg
Sodium bicarbonate	1 mEq/kg/dose IV/IO slowly	After adequate ventilation

**Flush with 5 mL of normal saline and follow with 5 ventilations.*

Table 4.
Pediatric resuscitation medications & doses.

5. Secondary survey

- The purpose of the secondary survey is to identify all injuries and perform a thorough & systematic head to toe examination. The injuries pointed out in the anatomical peculiarities section above should be especially looked for. Extreme vigilance in monitoring and re-evaluation must be ensured. Also research suggests that a third survey is one of the best ways to detect injuries that were missed during primary or secondary assessments [29–31].

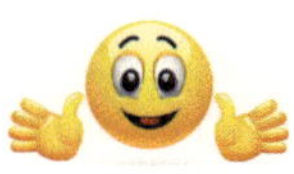

6. Extremity trauma and fracture biomechanics

- This needs special mention. Extremity fractures may initially be missed in a severely injured patient as clinicians attend to more life-threatening injuries.

- Modern war ballistics and blast injuries inflict devastating extremity injuries, violating soft tissue, bone, and neurovascular structures [32].

- Children suffer injuries different than that of adults, due to differences in their skeletal system. The important differences as compared to adults are (i) periosseous cartilage presence (ii) physes presence (iii) a thicker, stronger, and more osteogenic periosteum. This produces new bone called callus more rapidly and in greater amounts (iv) a disproportionately large head (v) pliable rib cage (vi) open epiphyseal plates (vii) low density and more porosity. The low density is due to lower mineral content and the increased porosity due to increased number of haversian canals and vascular channels.

These differences result in a comparatively lower modulus of elasticity and lower bending strength. The bone in children may fail either in tension or in compression. The fracture lines do not propagate as in adults, and hence less chances of comminuted fractures in children.

7. Burns

- Wartime burn care is important. Thermal injury historically constitutes approximately 5%–20% of conventional warfare casualties [33]. In a recent study of pediatric wartime admissions burns was the second leading cause of pediatric mortality at the Combat Support Hospital, & burns cases also had a high case fatality rate [5]. Thus burns care is essential, & expertise in care required for saving lives.

- Proper triage & treatment requires assessment of the extent and depth of the injury. Infants have thinner skin, therefore they get deep burns. The extent of burns is determined by the Wallace rule of nines in adults. In pediatric age group the Lund and Browder chart provides Body Surface Area (BSA) proportions at different ages, with decreasing percentage BSA for the head and increasing percentage BSA for the legs as the child ages (**Figure 1**). This is

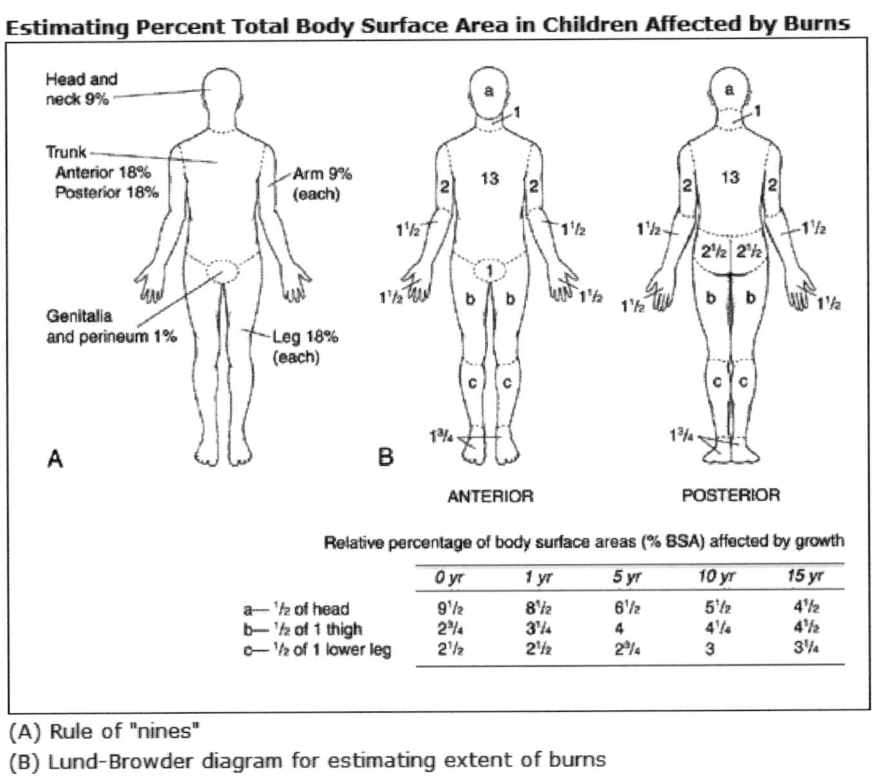

	0 yr	1 yr	5 yr	10 yr	15 yr
a— 1/2 of head	$9\frac{1}{2}$	$8\frac{1}{2}$	$6\frac{1}{2}$	$5\frac{1}{2}$	$4\frac{1}{2}$
b— 1/2 of 1 thigh	$2\frac{3}{4}$	$3\frac{1}{4}$	4	$4\frac{1}{4}$	$4\frac{1}{2}$
c— 1/2 of 1 lower leg	$2\frac{1}{2}$	$2\frac{1}{2}$	$2\frac{3}{4}$	3	$3\frac{1}{4}$

Figure 1.
The Lund and Browder chart. All numbers are percentages.

useful in pediatric burns. In near future we should be using newer imaging technologies like Forward-Looking Infra-Red (FLIR) for burn assessments [34].

- Children with burns of >15% of BSA should receive IV fluids, as in children there is risk of gastric distension with oral fluids. Several different formulas are used to calculate fluid requirements. Urine output remains the best indicator of volume status, with minimum target value of 1 mL/kg/hr. in children (in adults it is 0.5 mL/kg/hr). If carbon monoxide poisoning is suspected 100% oxygen should be administered.

8. Mental health

- Armed conflicts can adversely affect the mental health of children. Many mental disorders can occur, especially posttraumatic stress disorder (PTSD). A recent study has highlighted the need for intervention programs, for the detection, prevention, and treatment of PTSD symptoms for all children, regardless of exposure type, in areas affected by conflict [35].

- We must ensure proper psychological support in emergency, and always plan for psychological monitoring and rehabilitation.

9. Conclusions

- The combat casualty care being provided today is on the basis of experience in previous wars and the information generated by integrated research during and between conflicts. Continuation of such research is desirable. Research results refine our practices. All this will ensure ongoing progress and further improvements in the outcomes of both military and civilian casualties.

- A progressive outlook, proclivity to change opinion, & practice in the light of new developments will allow great advances to be achieved.

- The mortality and morbidity rates in pediatrics are considered to be the most important indicators of the health status of a community and level of living of people in general. If we are able to care for children in war also then it will be par excellence.

Acknowledgements

I'm indebted to all my teachers and seniors for inculcating best practices for results & inspiring better proficiency through research, in the march towards excellence in care of all children, at all places, and at all times.

Conflict of interest

"The authors declare no conflict of interest."

Thanks

Thankful to all the authors of references quoted for all the universally useful contributions in care of children.

Author details

Sunil Jain
Professor and Head, Department of Paediatrics, Command Hospital (Northern Command), India

*Address all correspondence to: sunil_jain700@rediff.com

References

[1] Russo RM, Neff LP. Pediatric Combat Trauma. Curr Trauma Rep. 2016; 2: 247–255. DOI 10.1007/s40719-016-0061-z

[2] Edwards MJ, Lustik M, Burnett MW, Eichelberger M. Pediatric inpatient humanitarian care in combat: Iraq and Afghanistan 2002 to 2012. J Am Coll Surg 2014; 218(5): 1018–23. doi: 10.1016/j.jamcollsurg.2013.12.050.

[3] Lundy JB, Swift CB, McFarland CC, Mahoney P, Perkins RM, Holcomb JB. A Descriptive Analysis of Patients Admitted to the Intensive Care Unit of the 10th Combat Support Hospital Deployed in Ibn Sina, Baghdad, Iraq, From Oct19, 2005 to Oct19, 2006. J Intensive Care Med. 2010; 25(3):156–62. doi: 10.1177/0885066609359588.

[4] Burnett MW, Spinella PC, Azarow KS, Callahan CW. Pediatric care as part of the US Army medical mission in the global war on terrorism in Afghanistan and Iraq, December 2001 to December 2004. Pediatrics. 2008; 121 (2): 261–5.

[5] Creamer KM, Edwards MJ, Shields CH, Thompson MW, Yu CE, Adelman W. Pediatric wartime admissions to US military combat support hospitals in Afghanistan and Iraq: learning from the first 2,000 admissions. J Trauma. 2009; 67(4): 762–8.

[6] Edwards MJ, Lustik M, Eichelberger MR, Elster E, Azarow K, Coppola C. Blast injury in children: an analysis from Afghanistan and Iraq, 2002–2010. J Trauma Acute Care Surg. 2012; 73(5): 1278–83.

[7] Haverkamp FJC, van Gennip L, Muhrbeck M, Veen H, Wladis A, Tan ECTH. Global surgery for paediatric casualties in armed conflict. World J Emerg Surg. 2019; 14: 55. doi: 10.1186/s13017-019-0275-9.

[8] Gale HL, Borgman MA, April MD, Schauer SG. Pediatric Trauma Patient Intensive Care Resource Utilization in U.S. Military Operations in Iraq and Afghanistan. Crit Care Explor. 2019; 1 (12): e0062. doi: 10.1097/CCE.0000000000000062.

[9] Lander A. Principles of paediatric surgery. In: Williams N, O'connell PR, McCaskie AW. editors Bailey & Loves Short Practice of Surgery 27th ed. Boca Raton FL: CRC Press; 2018. p 119–138.

[10] Matos RI, Holcomb JB, Callahan C, Spinella PC. Increased mortality rates of young children with traumatic injuries at a US army combat support hospital in Baghdad, Iraq, 2004. Pediatrics. 2008; 122(5): e959–66

[11] Butler FK. Two Decades of Saving Lives on the Battlefield: Tactical Combat Casualty Care Turns 20. Mil Med. 2017; 182(3): e1563-e1568. doi: 10.7205/MILMED-D-16-00214.

[12] Hamill J. Damage control surgery in children. Injury 2004; 35(7): 708–12.

[13] Westhorpe RN. The position of the larynx in children and its relationship to the ease of intubation. Anaesth Intense Care. 1987; 15: 384–8. doi: 10.1177/0310057X8701500405.

[14] Bendinelli C. Effects of land mines and unexploded ordnance on the pediatric population and comparison with adults in rural Cambodia. World J Surg. 2009; 33(5): 1070–4.

[15] Lesperance K, Martin MJ, Beekley AC, Steele SR The significance of penetrating gluteal injuries: an analysis of the Operation Iraqi Freedom experience. J Surg Educ. 2008; 65(1): 61–6

[16] Selbst SM, Fein JA, Osterhoudt K, Ho W. Medication errors in a pediatric

emergency department. Pediatr Emerg Care. 1999; 15(1): 1–4. doi: 10.1097/00006565-199902000-00001

[17] Cooper BR, Mahoney PF, Hodgetts TJ, Mellor A. Intra-osseous access (EZ-IO) for resuscitation: UK military combat experience. J R Army Med Corps. 2007; 153(4): 314–6.

[18] Talving P, Lustenberger T, Lam L, Inaba K, Mohseni S, Plurad D, et al. Coagulopathy after isolated severe traumatic brain injury in children. J Trauma. 2011;71(5): 1205–1210. doi: 10.1097/TA.0b013e31820d151d

[19] Leeper CM, Neal MD, McKenna C, Billiar T, Gaines BA. Principal component analysis of coagulation assays in severely injured children. Surgery. 2018; 163(4): 827–831. doi: 10.1016/j.surg.2017.09.031

[20] Leeper CM, Neal MD, Billiar TR, Sperry JL, Gaines BA. Overresuscitation with plasma is associated with sustained fibrinolysis shutdown and death in pediatric traumatic brain injury. J Trauma Acute Care Surg. 2018; 85(1): 12–17. doi:10.1097/TA.0000000000001836

[21] Shih AW, Al Khan S, Wang AY-H, Dawe P, Young PY, Greene A, et al. Systematic reviews of scores and predictors to trigger activation of massive transfusion protocols. J Trauma Acute Care Surg. 2019; 87(3): 717–729. doi:10.1097/TA.0000000000002372

[22] Ralston M, Hazinski MF, Zaritsky AL, Schexnayder SM, Kleinman ME, editors: *Pediatric advanced life support course guide and PALS provider manual: provider Manual*. American Heart Association. Dallas, TX: 2007.

[23] Teasdale G, Jennett B. Assessment of coma and impaired consciousness: a practical scale. Lancet. 1974; 2(7872): 81–84.

[24] Martin M, Oh J, Currier H, Tai N, Beekley A, Eckert M. An analysis of in-hospital deaths at a modern combat support hospital. J Trauma. 2009; 66(4 Suppl): S51–60; discussion S60–1.

[25] Roskind CG, Pryor II HI, Klein BL. Acute Care of Multiple Trauma. In: Kliegman RM, St. Geme JW, Blum NJ, Shah SS, Tasker RC, Wilson KM, et al editors. Nelson TB of Pediatrics. 21st ed. Philadelphia: Elsevier; 2020.

[26] Gilley M, Beno S. Damage control resuscitation in pediatric trauma. Curr Opin Pediatr. 2018; 30(3): 338–343. doi: 10.1097/MOP.0000000000000617.

[27] Gurney I. Paediatric casualties during OP TELIC. J R Army Med Corps. 2004;150(4): 270–2.

[28] Neff LP, Cannon JW, Charnock KM, Farmer DL, Borgman MA, Ricca RL. Elective pediatric surgical care in a forward deployed setting: What is feasible vs. what is reasonable. J Pediatr Surg 2016; 51(3): 409–15. doi: 10.1016/j.jpedsurg.2015.08.060.

[29] Soundappan SVS, Holland AJA, Cass DT: Role of an extended tertiary survey in detecting missed injuries in children. *J Trauma.* 2004; 57(1): 114–118.

[30] Halpern P, Arnold JL, Stok E, Ersoy G. Mass-casualty, terrorist bombings: Implications for emergency department and hospital emergency response (Part II). *Prehosp Disast Med.* 2003; 18(3): 235–241.

[31] Rutland-Brown W, Langlois JA, Nicaj L, Thomas, Jr. RG, Wilt SA, Bazarian JJ: Traumatic brain injuries after mass-casualty incidents: Lessons from the 11 September 2001 World Trade Center attacks. *Prehosp Disast Med.* 2007; 22(3): 57–164.

[32] Hawksworth JS, Stojadinovic A, Gage FA, Tadaki DK, Perdue PW,

Forsberg J, et al. Inflammatory biomarkers in combat wound healing. Ann Surg. 2009; 250(6): 1002–7.

[33] Cancio LC, Horvath EE, Barillo DJ, Kopchinski BJ, Charter KR, Montalvo AE, et al. Burn support for Operation Iraqi Freedom and related operations, 2003 to 2004. J Burn Care Rehabil. 2005; 26(2): 151–61.

[34] National Academies of Sciences, Engineering, and Medicine 2020. Army Combat Trauma Care in 2035: Proceedings of a Workshop in Brief. Washington, DC: The National Academies Press. https://doi.org/10.17226/25724.

[35] Eyüboglu M, Eyüboglu D, Sahin B, Fidan E. Posttraumatic stress disorder and psychosocial difficulties among children living in a conflict area of the Southeastern Anatolia region of Turkey. Indian J Psychiatry. 2019; 61(5): 496–502. doi: 10.4103/psychiatry.IndianJPsychiatry_165_18.

Chapter 5

Frostbite: A Conundrum in High Altitudes

Abhishek Kadian, Sachin Saini and Rajesh Khanna

Abstract

Cold injuries and its sequelae has for decades, been a relevant problem and an occupational hazard in the army, and continue to be so. These sequelae may hamper future operational capability of the soldier. Frostbite is also becoming more prevalent among the general population due to the increase in numbers of homeless people, along with an increasing participation in outdoor activities such as mountain hiking and skiing. Despite the advances in the field of medical sciences, frostbite management has remained constant and unchanged until recent years, when newer modalities of management have led to favourable, tissue-saving, outcomes. This chapter gives a background understanding of risk factors of frostbite and its pathophysiology and reviews the current evidence and latest frostbite management strategies. In addition, several adjunctive therapies and recent improvements in radiologic assessment of tissue viability provide new avenues of aggressive medical management and earlier surgical interventions.

Keywords: frostbite, rewarming, thrombolysis, prostacyclin, rTPA, gangrene, amputation, telemedicine, botulinum toxin

1. Introduction

Frostbite is defined as injury to body tissues caused by exposure to extreme cold, typically affecting the extremities and often involving only the skin, which initially becomes white and hard, but in severe cases resulting in gangrene of deeper tissues and loss of the affected parts [1].

The first physical evidence of frostbite injury dates back to 5000-year-old pre-Columbian mummy discovered in the Andes [2]. Baron Dominique Larrey, Napoleon's surgeon-in-chief during the infamous 1812 to 1813 retreat from Moscow, gave the first description of pathophysiology and management of frostbite [3]. Heavy bombers crew during World War II sustained more injuries due to high altitude frostbite than from all other causes combined [4]. Nazi-German Waffen during WWII had more than 10 mountain division of troops well-trained and adapted to operate cold of Arctic and mountains. Many of those mountain troops experienced devastating cold injuries [5].

Thus, the frostbite is a significant cause of long term irreversible morbidity in military medicine. Despite this, frostbite management has remained constant and unchanged. One of the most important factor often ignored is hypoxia related injuries associated with frost bite. The soldiers are often deployed at high altitude, face harsh climatic conditions in terms of exposure to cold and hypobaric hypoxia. Collectively, both these factors usually alter the course of certain conditions like cold related injuries at this height. However a number of novel therapies have been introduced in the last two decades which have led to promising, tissue-saving, outcomes.

The aim of this chapter is basic understanding of frostbite at high altitude conditions and incorporating latest frostbite management strategies to existing ones, both at prehospital levels and hospital levels, in order to maximise the tissue salvage of the patients.

2. Epidemiology

Frostbite continues to afflict modern militaries [6–8]. Within the civilian, most common is mountaineers.

The predisposing factors to cold injury include high altitude (above 17,000 feet), alcohol consumption, psychiatric illness, smoking, immobility, homelessness, unplanned exposure to cold with inadequate protection, contact with cold objects, previous history of cold injury, medical conditions like atherosclerosis, medications (eg, b-blockers), and working with equipment that uses refrigerant liquids and gases [9–14]. Also genetic factors like African American ethnicity, O group blood typing and angiotensin-converting enzyme DD allele may increase risk to cold injuries [7, 15, 16].

30–49 years are the Most susceptible age groups [17, 18]. Most common anatomic sites involved are hands and feets (90% of all recorded sites), others include ears, nose, cheeks and penis [17–22].

3. Pathophysiology

Two mechanisms that are apparently responsible for cold injury include direct cellular injury and progressive dermal ischemia.

3.1 Direct cellular injury

Due to freezing of tissue there is extracellular ice crystal formation, leading to electrolyte disturbances, intracellular dehydration and shrinkage leading to cell injury and death [23]. As temperature further falls, there is intracellular ice crystal formation, which expands leading to mechanical destruction of cells [24].

The body responds initially to it by alternating cycles of vasoconstriction and vasodilatation, known as "the hunting reaction" [25]. When vasodilatation occurs, there is reestablishment of blood flow, which is called thawing. The repeated freeze/thaw cycle causes most damage, and further leads to progressive thrombotic phase [24, 26, 27].

3.2 Progressive dermal ischemia

Progressive dermal ischemia is more severe than the direct cellular damage [28, 29]. **Figure 1** describes the events in progressive dermal ischemia [22].

Various studies have shown similarities in the progressive dermal ischemia due to frostbite and thermal burns [30, 31]. Blebs or blisters may develop secondary to vasodilatation, oedema, stasis and coagulation. Platelet and erythrocyte aggregates leads to thrombosis of the vessels in viable tissue. Local inflammatory response and associated injuries may cause increased compartment pressures [32]. Robson and Heggers found markedly elevated levels of prostaglandin F2a and thromboxane B2

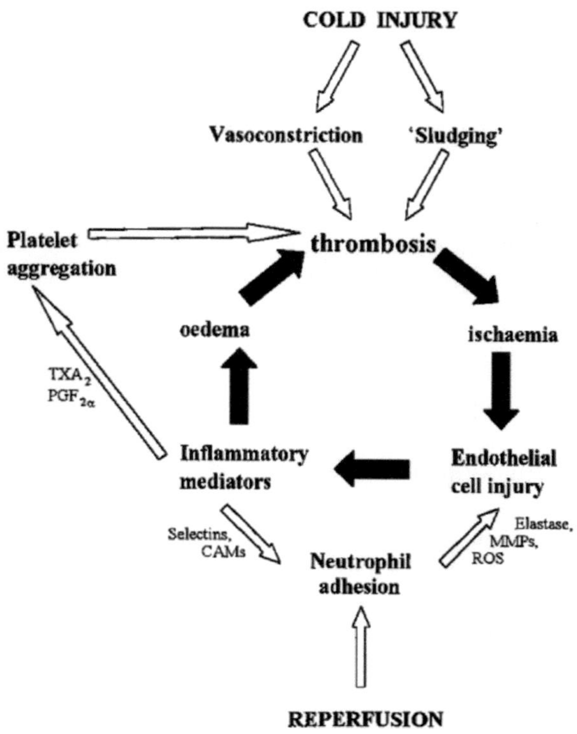

Figure 1.
Pathology of progressive dermal ischemia in frost bite. TXA_2, thromboxane A_2; PGF2α, prostaglandin $F_{2\alpha}$; CAM, cellular adhesions molecules; MMPs, matrix metalloproteinases; ROS, reactive oxygen species.

(a stable metabolite of thromboxane A2) in frostbite blister fluid [30, 33, 34]. Raine et al. demonstrated that prostaglandin and thromboxane inhibitors resulted in significantly improved tissue survival in rabbit ear frostbite [35]. Prostaglandin F2a (PGF2a) and thromboxane A2 (TXA2) cause platelet aggregation and thrombosis which results in ischaemia [32]. Thus there is significant role of the metabolites of arachidonic acid pathway as mediators of progressive dermal ischemia in burn and frostbite.

Other studies indicate the cell mediated inflammatory response which leads to progressive ischemia and tissue necrosis is similar to the response seen following ischemic/reperfusion injury [36]. The ischemic/reperfusion injury has been described as the paradoxical exacerbation of cellular dysfunction and death, following restoration of blood flow to previous ischaemic tissues [37]. During reperfusion, an inflammatory reaction occurs with neutrophilic aggregation and adhesion to endothelial cells leading to the production of free radicals [38]. Manson, *et al.* also suggested the role of free radicals in ischemia/reperfusion related tissue necrosis leading to frostbite injury [39].

Thrombosis, endothelial damage, intravascular sludging, inflammatory mediators, free radicals, neutrophil adhesion, platelet aggregation, reperfusion injury, and oedema all play a role in contributing to progressive dermal ischemia and leads to cell death [22, 30, 35, 36, 39, 40].

Frostbite is more common at high altitude than at sea level. As the altitude increases the maximum oxygen uptake falls thereby reducing the body's ability to produce heat, while dehydration, cold, the fall in plasma volume which occurs at high altitude and increased erythropoietin production all work to increase blood viscosity and reduce peripheral blood flow. This reduced peripheral perfusion due to hypoxia causes additive effect in pathophysiology of frostbite. A reduction in calorie intake also reduces insulating subcutaneous fat [39, 41]. Also, the blood microcirculation recovery after high altitude frostbite is significantly slower than the normal frostbite [42].

4. Clinical manifestations

Historically, the degrees classification has been favoured. It classifies frostbite into frostnip, first-degree, second-degree, third-degree, and fourth-degree frostbite depending on depth of injury [22]. This classifications fail to predict the extent of likely amputation levels and aid little in initial management.

Cauchy and colleagues [43] proposed a classification system for severity of frostbite cases, as depicted in **Table 1** (**Figure 2**). The advantage of this classification is that it gives an early prognostic indicator of bone and tissue loss and the likely anatomic level of loss. This grading system relies on isotope bone scanning. In the field, Cauchy and colleagues [44] suggest the use of portable Doppler or the clinical stigmata of soft tissue cyanosis as surrogate markers for amputation risk.

Initial symptoms include numbness and pale/bluish discolouration in the affected part. Following thawing, patient may complaint of throbbing pain and tingling sensation with/ without appearance of blisters (clear/hemorrhagic) in affected part. Long term sequelae includes cold insensitivity, sensory loss, hyperhidrosis [22], growth plate disturbances [25, 45], osteoarthritis [46], chronic pain [25], and hypertrophic calcification [47]. There are few case reports of frostbite with extensive limb involvement showing rare presentation as acute compartment syndrome and increasing rhabdomyolysis. There was no other clear aetiology of rhabdomyolysis in these cases and they required compartment release [48].

On physical examination favourable prognostic indicators include normal skin colour, sensation to pinprick, blisters with clear fluid and the ability of the skin to deform under direct pressure. Poor prognostic indicators include non blanching cyanosis, hemorrhagic blisters and hard, non deforming skin [22].

Chilblains is a self limiting, mild form of cold injury in which there is appearance of red, itchy lesions on the limbs on exposure to temperature above freezing point. Tissue loss is rare. It is managed conservatively by limb elevation and application of moisturising lotions [22].

Grade	Extent of initial lesion day 0	Bone scan, day 2	Blisters at day 2	Prognosis at day 2
1	No lesion	Unnecessary	No blisters	No amputation
2	Lesion distal phalanx only	Reduced radiotracer uptake	Clear blister fluid	Tissue excision
3	Lesion distal, inter-and proximal phalanx	No radiotracer uptake on digit	Hemorrhagic blister fluid	Bone amputation of digit
4	Lesion in carpel/tarsal	No tracer uptake in carpal/ tarsal	Hemorrhagic blisters carpal/ tarsal	Bone amputation of limb

After Cauchy et al. [43].
The initial assessment on arrival in hospital, day 0, is made after rapid rewarming.

Table 1.
Classification scheme for severity of frostbite injuries.

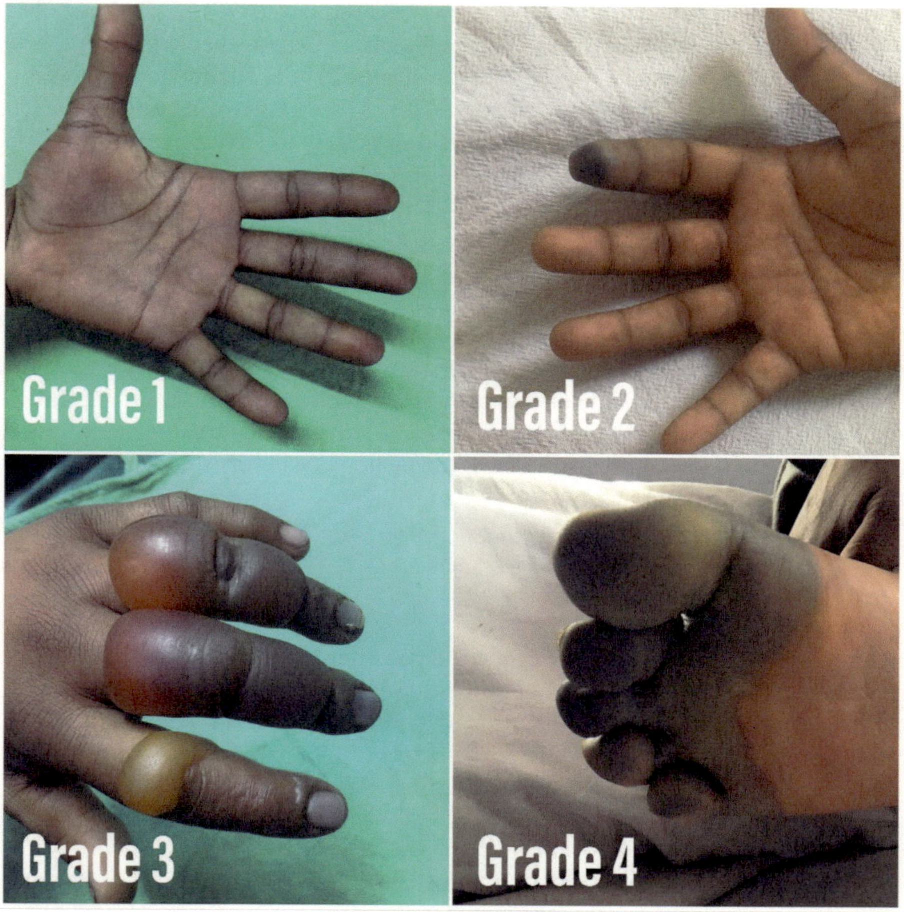

Figure 2.
Grades of frostbite.

5. Radiology

In order to provide early assessment of tissue viability and management several radiological techniques can be used like bone scanning, magnetic resonance angiography (MRA), and angiography.

Technecium 99 (99 Tc) triple-phase bone scanning has become the standard imaging study when used at day 2 post cold injury [43, 49–51]. It helps to assess tissue viability but fails to show clear-cut soft tissue demarcation. However, MRA is often easier to access and allows direct visualisation of thrombosed vessels and may show a clearer demarcation of viable and ischemic tissues. Therefore some authors advocate MRA as superior technique [52, 53]. Digital subtraction angiography can be performed on individuals who are being considered for thrombolysis. It visualises vessel patency but do not sufficiently clarifies the level of viability [49, 54].

6. Prevention

As "prevention is better than cure" it is the responsibility of commanders, team leaders, individuals, and companies/employers who place individuals in at-risk areas. The following preventive measures should be adopted: 1) maintain adequate hydration and nutritional status; 2) use multilayered clothing preferably wool or synthetics such as polypropylene as these materials insulate even when wet. Also avoid constricting items like tight cramp on straps. Proper fitting boots should be worn. Mittens are preferable to finger gloves; 3) avoid sweating and prolonged immobility; 4) Avoid fatigue and one should not climb in adverse weather conditions; 5) buddy care system should be followed and one should daily inspect foot to look for any signs of cold injury; 6) ensure beneficial behavioural responses to changing climatic conditions like avoiding alcohol and smoking. Alcohol causes cutaneous vasodilatation which gives temporary warmth but actually causes greater heat loss. Similarly, nicotine in cigarette causes vasoconstriction and thereby aggravates cellular hypoxia [55]; 7) do not touch metallic objects in extreme cold or in moderate cold if wet; 8) leaders/commanders must ensure that all are fit, trained, and capable of operating in proposed location/climate; this should take into account the co-morbidities and current medications; and 9) a thorough evacuation and medical plan must be in place before departure; this must include communications.

7. Management

Before evaluating the patient one should consider that once the boots are removed, the swelling may occur, so prevent redonning of boots. Also, freeze–thaw–freeze cycles must be avoided; therefore, only consider rewarming if this can be avoided. It may be better to walk out on a frozen foot.

7.1 Prehospital management

It is treatment by persons with limited medical background.

7.1.1 Basic care

One should thoroughly assess the patient as he may be having concurrent hypothermia. Remove all wet clothing and jewellery. Provide general warmth. Rehydrate the individual with adequate warm fluids. Avoid smoking and alcohol.

7.1.2 Rewarming

Immerse the affected part in water at 40 °C to 42 °C with a mild antibacterial agent like providone-iodine [25, 35, 54, 56]. If a thermometer is not available then first the unaffected limb should be placed in water for at least 30 seconds to ensure that the water is not too hot as the affected limb will have impaired temperature sensation. Twice-daily baths are recommended and redressing should be done every 12 to 24 hours [57]. Avoid mechanical trauma to the affected part. Do not rub or applying dry heat (heat pads) to frozen tissue. Thawing is complete only when the red/purple and pliable texture of affected part is achieved [25, 58]. Once thawing is complete, the limb should be allowed to air dry. Thereafter keep affected limb completely warm. Avoid re-exposure. Elevate the affected limb to reduce oedema [57].

7.1.3 Medications

Cold-injured part is a tetanus prone wound; therefore follow standard tetanus toxoid guidelines [23, 25, 59]. Give ibuprofen 12 mg/kg twice a day up to a maximum of 2400 mg/d, for analgesia and to reduce inflammation (unless contraindicated) [49]. It supersedes aspirin as aspirin inhibits prostaglandins, some of which are beneficial to healing [23–25]. *Aloe vera* is a topical inhibitor of thromboxane; [35] apply to the affected part and cover with a dry dressing. Blisters indicate thawing [57]. Do not aspirate or de-roof them in the field. Avoid circumferential dressings. Give tablet oxpentifylline 400 mg thrice a day; studies have shown that with *Aloe vera*, oxpentifylline leads to 30% improvement in overall tissue survival [60]. The role of prophylactic antibiotics is controversial [57], it is generally reserved if signs of infection and specific complications develop [22]. The doctors at forward location should seek expert help via telemedicine.

7.1.4 Portable recompression bag and oxygenation

Portable recompression bag simulate physiological "descent" and there is increase in SpO2 [44, 61]. It can be used as an adjunct, provided patient is fully conscious and it should not delay evacuation. Supplemental oxygen may be beneficial at high altitudes posts [44] with an aim to maintain SpO2 greater than 90% [57].

7.2 Hospital management

Once the patient is transferred to a hospital take detailed history including onset of injury (<24 hours or > 24 hours ago), mechanism of injury, climatic conditions at time of injury, any freeze–thaw–freeze events, and in-field treatment. Reassess the patient and affected parts thoroughly. Keep the individual in a warm room. Remove all jewellery if not removed previously. Rehydrate the patient with warm fluids and give high-protein, high-calorie diets [62]. Follow rewarming principles as described above.

Give tetanus toxoid, if not given previously. Continue oral ibuprofen and oxypentifylline as described above. Analgesics may be required on an individual basis (paracetamol, tramadol, opiates). The role of prophylactic antibiotics in frostbite is controversial [17]. However, systemic antibiotics must be commenced in proven infection as guided by skin swab culture sensitivity [63].

Blisters give an indication to the depth of injury. White/clear blisters indicate superficial injury and contains high levels of prostaglandin $F_{2\alpha}$ and thromboxane A_2 [30]; therefore aspiration may be beneficial. However, few authors have advocated that clear blisters should be left intact, and de-roofing may result in increased susceptibility to opportunistic infections [64]. Hemorrhagic blisters indicate structural damage to reticular dermis; many authors advocate them to be left intact due to risk of desiccation [18, 24]. The Wilderness Medical Society guidelines advise drainage of white/clear blisters and to leave hemorrhagic blisters alone [57].

Dressing of the affected areas should be done 12 or 24 hourly and the affected part should be splinted and elevated. Dressing should be non constrictive and loose with padding between the digits. Apply *Aloe vera* cream to the affected part. Bespoke safety footwear should be worn during the demarcation period.

Take photograph of the affected part on admission and subsequently every alternate day. If facilities are available one should consider imaging like bone scanning, magnetic resonance angiography (MRA), and angiography. It offers prognostic information and guide management.

7.3 Adjunctive therapies

The following adjunctive therapies have been described recently.

7.3.1 Low molecular weight dextran

It is a grade 2C recommendation for use when thrombolytics or iloprost are not going to be used. However, there are no clinical trials to prove its role and also it can cause anaphylaxis; [44] We do not recommend it.

7.3.2 Anticoagulation

Post thawing, thrombosis is seen to occur in superficial dermal plexus. Therefore anticoagulation with heparin may have a role in frostbite but there is no evidence in literature for it [22, 56, 65]. So it is not recommended as monotherapy.

7.3.3 Hyperbaric oxygen

Hyperbaric oxygen therapy (HBOT) increases oxygen delivery to the tissues provided there must be a patent vasculature [57]. However, it could help during rewarming phase and at high altitude (usually >4000 meters) when SpO2 is less than 90% [66]. It is suggested that immediately after rapid rewarming, do HBOT for 1 hour. Thereafter, it can be repeated every 3 hours during the first 12 hours while the patient is awaiting evacuation [44, 61].

7.3.4 Sympathetic nerve blocks

Many studies have shown that sympathetic nerve block in upper limb causes vasodilation, raised skin temperature and pain relief [67]. Its role in frost bite cases is mixed [68–71]. However, it is possible that very early intervention with sympathetic blockade in the field may be more effective. Chandral et al. described a technique for giving peripheral nerve block [69]. The same technique was used by Pasquier et al. in field area for managing grade 2 frostbite in bilateral hand [72]. He performed bilateral wrist block using 0.5% ropivacaine. There was good recovery without amputation. Taylor et al. used continuous epidural anaesthesia for managing frostbite cases of lower limbs [73]. Therefore, for grade 2–4 frostbite cases following thawing, which are limited to hands, distal volar forearm nerve block may be considered. Similarly for lower limbs, continuous epidural catheter may be considered for analgesia and vasodilation.

7.3.5 Thrombolysis and vasodilation

Thrombolytic agents have been used for reversing microvascular thrombosis and restoring blood flow. Thrombolysis using streptokinase, urokinase or recombinant tissue plasminogen activator (rTPA) has resulted in reduced amputation rates [14, 49, 74, 75]. Limited data suggest that rTPA in frostbite is most effective when used within 6 to 24 hours of rewarming [14, 44, 49, 74, 76]. However, studies have shown that ilioprost (a synthetic analogue of prostacyclin PGI2) has better safety profile than rTPA and is most effective up to 48 hours after rewarming [77, 78]. In field location, grade 2 to 4 frostbite may result in tissue loss if not treated. Therefore, trained medicine specialist can initiate treatment with ilioprost or rTPA, considering their contraindications and complications, for grade 2 to 4 frostbite as per dosage and considerations given in **Tables 2** and **3** respectively [44].

Administration and monitoring	Dilute 1 vial 0.5 mL iloprost in 24.5 mL NaCl 9% Syringe pump: 25 mL - speed: 1 mL/ h for 30 minutes, then 2 mL/h for 30 minutes, then 3 mL/h for 30 minutes, then 4 mL/h for weight < 75 kg or 5 mL/h for weight > 75 kg Continue until 25 mL is delivered; all patients receive 1 vial Monitor HR and BP every 30 minutes
Complications and their management	In case of side effects decrease to previous lower step If systolic BP <90 mmHg decrease to lower step
Contraindications	Hypotension, hypersensitivity, pulmonary edema, cardiac arrhythmia, active ulcer disease, major trauma; unknown effects on pregnancy
Precautions	Anticipate nausea and vomiting, pain and hypotension; keep patient supine

HR, heart rate; BP, blood pressure.

Table 2.
Protocol for intravenous prostacyclin.

Administration	Weight < 67 kg: 15 mg IV bolus, then 0.75 mg/kg over 30 minutes, then 0.35 mg/kg over next 60 minutes
Ideally given with a portable syringe pump	Weight > 67 kg: 15 mg IV bolus, then 50 mg over 30 minutes, then 35 mg over next 60 minutes. Total not to exceed 100 mg Heparin after bolus
Contraindications	Recent trauma, bleeding diathesis, stroke within 3 months, on anticoagulants, hypersensitivity; BP >180 mmHg systolic or 110 mmHg diastolic
Precautions	High altitude: HAPE or HACE, retinal haemorrhage, gastritis
Complications and their management	Bleeding: stop infusion, haemostasis if possible, consider tranexamic acid Angioedema: stop infusion, antihistamine, corticosteroids

rTPA, recombinant tissue plasminogen activator; IV, intravenous; BP, blood pressure; HAPE: high altitude pulmonary edema; HACE: high altitude cerebral edema.

Table 3.
Protocol for intravenous rTPA.

7.3.6 Botulinum toxin

Botulinum toxin is produced by *Clostridium botulinum*. Botulinum toxin type A (BTX-A) blocks the release of the neurotransmitter acetylcholine at the motor end plate terminals, thereby inhibiting the smooth muscle vasoconstriction [79]. It also blocks the transmission of norepinephrine and prevents sympathetic vasoconstriction of vascular smooth muscle [80].

In addition it causes reduction in pain by blocking recruitment of specific α2- adrenoreceptors, which decreases the activity of chronically upregulated C-fibre nociceptors [81]. Also the effects last for 3–4 months. Norheim et al. used BTX-A injections at the neurovascular bundles in the palm of each hand at the level of the metacarpophalangeal joints in a patient with frostbite sequelae [82]. Their study shows that BTX-A has positive effects on skin perfusion, cold hypersensitivity and pain. They speculated that early treatment of frostbite sequelae with BTX-A may be advantageous.

7.4 Surgical treatment

The general dictum is "Frostbite in January, amputate in July" [25]. Avoid immediate or early amputation. Wait till demarcation is complete to maximise functional outcome [56]. It may take 3 months. However, in cases of wet gangrene or spreading sepsis, early amputation may be unavoidable [83, 84]. For such cases, using MRA/99Tc triple-phase bone scanning is useful in planning the site of amputation [63]. Some authors advocate that coverage with vascularised tissue and free tissue transfer, rather than autograft improves the viability of injured bone, tendon or nerve, if early surgical intervention is done [85, 86].

In case patient develops compartment syndrome, escharotomy or fasciotomy may be indicated in the early phase [25, 56].

8. Conclusion

For the military, frostbite sequelae constitute an occupational injury with a major career impact. These sequelae may compromise future operational capability of the soldier. This chapter highlights simple and effective treatment steps that all clinicians can perform through every echelon of care and thereby reduce the period in which the patient is unable to perform his or her normal duties as a soldier in a cold environment.

Conflict of interest

No potential conflict of interest was reported by the authors.

Author details

Abhishek Kadian*, Sachin Saini and Rajesh Khanna
Army College of Medical Sciences, New Delhi, India

*Address all correspondence to: kadianabhishek@gmail.com

References

[1] Dictionary, O.E., *"art, n.1"*. 2016: Oxford University Press.

[2] Post, P.W. and D.D. Donner, *Frostbite in a pre-Columbian mummy.* Am J Phys Anthropol, 1972. **37**(2): p. 187-191.

[3] baron Larrey, D.J., *Memoirs of Military Surgery, and Campaigns of the French Armies, on the Rhine, in Corsica, Catalonia, Egypt, and Syria; at Boulogne, Ulm, and Austerlitz; in Saxony, Prussia, Poland, Spain, and Austria*. Vol. 1. 1814: Joseph Cushing, 6, North Howard street.

[4] Dembert, M.L., L.M. Dean, and E.M. Noddin, *Cold weather morbidity among United States navy and marine corps personnel.* Military medicine, 1981. **146**(11): p. 771-775.

[5] Dupuy, R.E. and T.N. Dupuy, *The Harper Encyclopedia of Military History, 4ª edição*. 1993, Nova York: HarperCollins Publishers.

[6] Heil, K.M., E. Oakley, and A. Wood, *British Military freezing cold injuries: a 13-year review.* Journal of the Royal Army Medical Corps, 2016. **162**(6): p. 413-418.

[7] DeGroot, D.W., et al., *Epidemiology of US Army cold weather injuries, 1980-1999.* Aviation, space, and environmental medicine, 2003. **74**(5): p. 564-570.

[8] Moran, D.S., et al., *Hypothermia and local cold injuries in combat and non-combat situations—the Israeli experience.* Aviation, space, and environmental medicine, 2003. **74**(3): p. 281-284.

[9] Mulgrew, S., et al., *Cold finger: urban frostbite in the UK.* BMJ case reports, 2013. **2013**: p. bcr1120115167.

[10] Sever, C., et al., *Unusual hand frostbite caused by refrigerant liquids and gases.* Turkish Journal of Trauma and Emergency Surgery, 2010. **16**(5): p. 433-438.

[11] Wegener, E., K. Barraza, and S. Das, *Severe frostbite caused by Freon gas.* Southern medical journal, 1991. **84**(9): p. 1143-1146.

[12] Mäkinen, T.M., et al., *Occurrence of frostbite in the general population–work-related and individual factors.* Scandinavian journal of work, environment & health, 2009: p. 384-393.

[13] Rintamäki, H., *Predisposing factors and prevention of frostbite.* International journal of circumpolar health, 2000. **59**(2): p. 114-121.

[14] Bruen, K.J., et al., *Reduction of the incidence of amputation in frostbite injury with thrombolytic therapy.* Archives of surgery, 2007. **142**(6): p. 546-553.

[15] Giesbrecht, G.G. and J.A. Wilkerson, *Hypothermia, frostbite and other cold injuries: prevention, survival, rescue, and treatment*. 2006: The Mountaineers Books.

[16] Kamikomaki, N., *A climber with the DD ACE allele developed frostbite despite taking more than adequate measures against cold on Mount Everest.* High altitude medicine & biology, 2007. **8**(2): p. 167-168.

[17] Valnicek, S.M., L.R. Chasmar, and J.B. Clapson, *Frostbite in the prairies: a 12-year review.* Plastic and reconstructive surgery, 1993. **92**(4): p. 633-641.

[18] Pulla, R., L. Pickard, and T. Carnett, *Frostbite: an overview with case presentations.* The Journal of foot and ankle surgery: official publication of the American College of Foot and Ankle Surgeons, 1994. **33**(1): p. 53-63.

[19] Lehmuskallio, E., et al., *Frostbite of the face and ears: epidemiological study of risk factors in Finnish conscripts.* Bmj, 1995. **311**(7021): p. 1661-1663.

[20] Hermann, G., et al., *The problem of frostbite in civilian medical practice.* The Surgical clinics of North America, 1963. **43**: p. 519.

[21] Rosen, L., et al., *Local cold injuries sustained during military service in the Norwegian Army.* Arctic medical research, 1991. **50**(4): p. 159-165.

[22] Murphy, J.V., et al., *Frostbite: pathogenesis and treatment.* Journal of Trauma and Acute Care Surgery, 2000. **48**(1): p. 171.

[23] Bracker, M., *Environmental and thermal injury.* Clinics in sports medicine, 1992. **11**(2): p. 419-436.

[24] Heggers, J.P., et al., *Experimental and clinical observations on frostbite.* Annals of emergency medicine, 1987. **16**(9): p. 1056-1062.

[25] Britt, L.D., W.H. Dascombe, and A. Rodriguez, *New horizons in management of hypothermia and frostbite injury.* Surgical Clinics of North America, 1991. **71**(2): p. 345-370.

[26] Washburn, B.F., *What it is. How to prevent it. Emergency treatment.* N. Engl. J. Med, 1962. **266**: p. 974-989.

[27] MAZUR, P. *Causes of injury in frozen and thawed cells*. in *Federation proceedings*. 1965.

[28] Auerbach, P., P. Hackett, and R. Roach, *High Altitude Medicine and Physiology.* Wilderness Medicine. 6th ed. Philadelphia, PA: Elsevier Mosby, 2012.

[29] VanGelder, C.M. and R.L. Sheridan, *Freezing soft tissue injury from propane gas.* Journal of Trauma and Acute Care Surgery, 1999. **46**(2): p. 355-356.

[30] Robson, M.C. and J.P. Heggers, *Evaluation of hand frostbite blister fluid as a clue to pathogenesis.* The Journal of hand surgery, 1981. **6**(1): p. 43-47.

[31] McCauley, R.L., et al., *Frostbite injuries: a rational approach based on the pathophysiology.* The Journal of trauma, 1983. **23**(2): p. 143-147.

[32] Grieve, A., et al., *A Clinical Review of the Management of Frostbite.* Journal of the Royal Army Medical Corps, 2011. **157**(1): p. 73-78.

[33] Heggers, J.P., et al., *Evaluation of burn blister fluid.* Plastic and reconstructive surgery, 1980. **65**(6): p. 798-804.

[34] Heggers, J.P., et al., *Histological demonstration of prostaglandins and thromboxanes in burned tissue.* Journal of Surgical Research, 1980. **28**(2): p. 110-117.

[35] Raine, T., et al. *Anti-prostaglandins and anti-thromboxanes for treatment of frostbite*. in *Surgical Forum*. 1980. AMER COLL SURGEONS 54 EAST ERIE ST, CHICAGO, IL 60611.

[36] Mohr, W.J., K. Jenabzadeh, and D.H. Ahrenholz, *Cold injury.* Hand clinics, 2009. **25**(4): p. 481-496.

[37] Cowled, P. and R. Fitridge, *Pathophysiology of reperfusion injury.* Mechanisms of Vascular Disease: A Reference Book for Vascular Specialists [Internet], 2011.

[38] Zook, N., et al., *Microcirculatory studies of frostbite injury.* Annals of plastic surgery, 1998. **40**(3): p. 246-253; discussion 254.

[39] Manson, P.N., et al., *Evidence for an early free radical-mediated reperfusion injury in frostbite.* Free Radical Biology and Medicine, 1991. **10**(1): p. 7-11.

[40] Kulka, J.P., *Microcirculatory impairment as a factor in inflammatory*

tissue damage. Annals of the New York Academy of Sciences, 1964. **116**(3): p. 1018-1044.

[41] Gautier, H., et al., *Hypoxia-induced changes in shivering and body temperature.* Journal of Applied Physiology, 1987. **62**(6): p. 2477-2484.

[42] JIAO, M.-k., et al., *Difference in blood microcirculation recovery between normal frostbite and high-altitude frostbite.* Medical Journal of Chinese People's Liberation Army, 2017. **42**(1): p. 66-69.

[43] Cauchy, E., et al., *Retrospective study of 70 cases of severe frostbite lesions: a proposed new classification scheme.* Wilderness & environmental medicine, 2001. **12**(4): p. 248-255.

[44] Cauchy, E., et al., *A new proposal for management of severe frostbite in the austere environment.* Wilderness & environmental medicine, 2016. **27**(1): p. 92-99.

[45] Reed, M., *Growth disturbances in the hands following thermal injuries in children. 2. Frostbite.* Canadian Association of Radiologists journal= Journal l'Association canadienne des radiologistes, 1988. **39**(2): p. 95-99.

[46] Rompe, G., *Unilateral finger polyarthrosis as a late sequel of frostbite.* Zeitschrift fur Orthopadie und ihre Grenzgebiete, 1988. **126**(3): p. 358-360.

[47] Larson, P., M. Weinstock, and R. Welch, *Calcification of the auricular cartilage: a case report and literature review.* Cutis, 1992. **50**(1): p. 55-57.

[48] Brandão, R.A., et al., *Acute compartment syndrome of the foot due to frostbite: literature review and case report.* The Journal of Foot and Ankle Surgery, 2018. **57**(2): p. 382-387.

[49] Handford, C., et al., *Frostbite: a practical approach to hospital management.* Extreme physiology & medicine, 2014. **3**(1): p. 7.

[50] Cauchy, E., et al., *The role of bone scanning in severe frostbite of the extremities: a retrospective study of 88 cases.* European journal of nuclear medicine, 2000. **27**(5): p. 497-502.

[51] Mehta, R.C. and M.A. Wilson, *Frostbite injury: prediction of tissue viability with triple-phase bone scanning.* Radiology, 1989. **170**(2): p. 511-514.

[52] Barker, J.R., et al., *Magnetic resonance imaging of severe frostbite injuries.* Annals of plastic surgery, 1997. **38**(3): p. 275-279.

[53] Raman, S., Z. Jamil, and J. Cosgrove, *Magnetic resonance angiography unmasks frostbite injury.* Emergency Medicine Journal, 2011. **28**(5): p. 450-450.

[54] Purdue, G.F. and J.L. Hunt, *Cold injury: a collective review.* The Journal of burn care & rehabilitation, 1986. **7**(4): p. 331-342.

[55] Nagpal, B. and R. Sharma, *Cold injuries: The chill within.* Medical Journal, Armed Forces India, 2004. **60**(2): p. 165.

[56] McCauley, R.L., et al., *Frostbite and other cold-induced injuries.* Wilderness Medicine: Management of Wilderness and Environmental Emergencies. 3rd ed. St Louis, MO: Mosby, 1995: p. 129-145.

[57] McIntosh, S.E., et al., *Wilderness Medical Society practice guidelines for the prevention and treatment of frostbite: 2014 update.* Wilderness & environmental medicine, 2014. **25**(4): p. S43-S54.

[58] Fritz, R. and D. Perrin, *Cold exposure injuries: prevention and treatment.* Clinics in sports medicine, 1989. **8**(1): p. 111-128.

[59] Vogel, J. and A. Dellon, *Frostbite injuries of the hand.* Clinics in plastic surgery, 1989. **16**(3): p. 565-576.

[60] Miller, M.B. and P.J. Koltai, *Treatment of experimental frostbite with pentoxifylline and aloe vera cream.* Archives of Otolaryngology–Head & Neck Surgery, 1995. **121**(6): p. 678-680.

[61] Cauchy, E., et al., *Portable hyperbaric chamber and management of hypothermia and frostbite: an evident utilization.* High altitude medicine & biology, 2014. **15**(1): p. 95-96.

[62] Kiss, T.L., *Critical care for frostbite.* Critical Care Nursing Clinics, 2012. **24**(4): p. 581-591.

[63] Handford, C., O. Thomas, and C.H. Imray, *Frostbite.* Emergency Medicine Clinics, 2017. **35**(2): p. 281-299.

[64] Hallam, M.-J., S. Lo, and C. Imray, *Frostbite*, in *Skin Necrosis*. 2015, Springer. p. 61-69.

[65] Schumacker, H.B., et al., *Studies in experimental frostbite: I. The effect of heparin in preventing gangrene.* Surgery, 1947. **22**(6): p. 900-909.

[66] Imray, C., et al., *Cold damage to the extremities: frostbite and non-freezing cold injuries.* Postgraduate medical journal, 2009. **85**(1007): p. 481-488.

[67] Hermanns, H., et al., *Skin temperature after interscalene brachial plexus blockade.* Regional anesthesia and pain medicine, 2007. **32**(6): p. 481-487.

[68] Calder, K., et al., *Bupivacaine digital blocks: how long is the pain relief and temperature elevation?* Plastic and reconstructive surgery, 2013. **131**(5): p. 1098-1104.

[69] Chandran, G.J., et al., *The hyperthermic effect of a distal volar forearm nerve block: a possible treatment of acute digital frostbite injuries?* Plastic and reconstructive surgery, 2010. **126**(3): p. 946-950.

[70] Shapovalov, K., E. Burdinskiĭ, and A. Stepanov, *Optimization of the components of regulation of vascular tone and microcirculatory hemostasis during prolonged regional block in local cold injury.* Anesteziologiia i reanimatologiia, 2008(3): p. 20-22.

[71] Syposs, T., et al., *Management of frostbite of the lower limbs by continuous epidural blockade.* Orvosi hetilap, 1986. **127**(1): p. 27-30.

[72] Pasquier, M., et al., *Pre-hospital wrist block for digital frostbite injuries.* High altitude medicine & biology, 2012. **13**(1): p. 65-66.

[73] Taylor, M.S., *Lumbar epidural sympathectomy for frostbite injuries of the feet.* Military medicine, 1999. **164**(8): p. 566-567.

[74] Twomey, J.A., G.L. Peltier, and R.T. Zera, *An open-label study to evaluate the safety and efficacy of tissue plasminogen activator in treatment of severe frostbite.* Journal of Trauma and Acute Care Surgery, 2005. **59**(6): p. 1350-1355.

[75] Lo, T.C., et al., *Combined radiation therapy and 5-fluorouracil for advanced squamous cell carcinoma of the oral cavity and oropharynx: a randomized study.* AJR Am J Roentgenol, 1976. **126**(2): p. 229-235.

[76] Johnson, A.R., et al., *Efficacy of intravenous tissue plasminogen activator in frostbite patients and presentation of a treatment protocol for frostbite patients.* Foot & ankle specialist, 2011. **4**(6): p. 344-348.

[77] Cauchy, E., B. Cheguillaume, and E. Chetaille, *A controlled trial of a prostacyclin and rt-PA in the treatment of severe frostbite.* New England Journal of Medicine, 2011. **364**(2): p. 189-190.

[78] Groechenig, E., *Treatment of frostbite with iloprost.* The Lancet, 1994. **344**(8930): p. 1152-1153.

[79] Fabregat, G., et al., *Subcutaneous and perineural botulinum toxin type A for neuropathic pain: a descriptive review.* The Clinical journal of pain, 2013. **29**(11): p. 1006-1012.

[80] Van Beek, A.L., et al., *Management of vasospastic disorders with botulinum toxin A.* Plastic and reconstructive surgery, 2007. **119**(1): p. 217-226.

[81] Morris, J.L., P. Jobling, and I.L. Gibbins, *Differential inhibition by botulinum neurotoxin A of cotransmitters released from autonomic vasodilator neurons.* American Journal of Physiology-Heart and Circulatory Physiology, 2001. **281**(5): p. H2124-H2132.

[82] Norheim, A.J., et al., *A new treatment for frostbite sequelae; Botulinum toxin.* International journal of circumpolar health, 2017. **76**(1): p. 1273677.

[83] Andrew, J., *Life and limb: a true story of tragedy and survival*. 2003: Portrait.

[84] Mills, J.W., *Frostbite. A discussion of the problem and a review of an Alaskan experience.* Alaska medicine, 1973. **15**(2): p. 27-47.

[85] Greenwald, D., B. Cooper, and L. Gottlieb, *An algorithm for early aggressive treatment of frostbite with limb salvage directed by triple-phase scanning.* Plastic and reconstructive surgery, 1998. **102**(4): p. 1069-1074.

[86] Izmaĭlov, G., et al., *Treatment of deep burns and frostbite of the hand and fingers.* Vestnik khirurgii imeni II Grekova, 1988. **141**(9): p. 80-82.